VEGAN COOKING

50 MEATLESS FAVORITES. MADE WITH PLANTS.

VIRGINIA FARMVILLE

TABLE OF CONTENTS

---- BREAKFAST ----

---- LUNCH ----

---- DINNER ----

---- SNACKS ----

---- DESSERTS ----

Breakfast

OVERNIGHT OATS

Overnight oats, a delicious, healthy, and nutritious breakfast or snack. It's ready in just 10 minutes with only 7 ingredients, and great to eat on the go!

MAKES 2 SERVING/ TOTAL TIME 10 MINUTE

INGREDIENTS

3/4 cup rolled oats (90 g), gluten-free if needed

1 tbsp chia seeds

1 tbsp maple syrup (optional)

1/2 tsp vanilla extract (optional)

1 cup milk of your choice (250 ml), I used unsweetened soy milk

Almond butter or peanut butter (optional)

Fresh blueberries (optional)

METHOD

STEP 1

Add all the ingredients into a jar (except the almond or peanut butter and the blueberries), stir, cover, and refrigerate overnight or for at least 4 hours.

Give it a good stir before serving and add more milk if needed.

STEP 2

Customize it with any kind of fresh fruit, dried fruits, nuts, seeds, or any other topping like ground cinnamon, cocoa powder, ground ginger, dark chocolate, shredded coconut, or matcha tea.

Keep the leftovers in a closed jar in the fridge for up to 3-4 days.

NUTRITION VALUE

177 KJ Energy, 7.2g fat, 0.9g saturated fat, 6.1g fiber, 8.3g protein, 19.9g carbs.

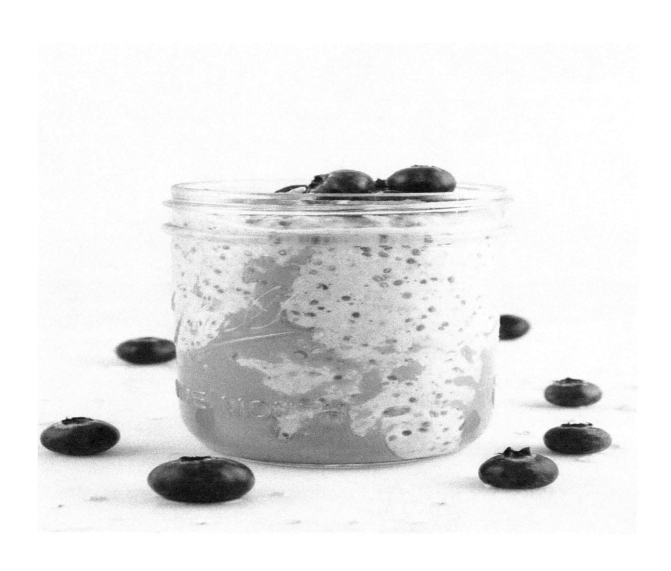

ECHINACEA AND VEGETABLE JUICE

Ward off cold and flu viruses by drinking this mixture of vegetable juice and echinacea tea daily- the vegies contain anti-oxidants and vitamin C, while echinacea boosts immune function.

MAKES 2 SERVING/ TOTAL TIME 15 MINUTE

INGREDIENTS

1 echinacea tea bag

80ml (1/3 cup) boiling water

2 large carrots, peeled, topped

1 red capsicum, halved, deseeded, thickly sliced

1 lime, peeled

Ice cubes (optional), to serve

METHOD

STEP 1

Place the tea bag in a small heatproof bowl and pour over boiling water. Set aside for 10 minutes to infuse.

STEP 2

Meanwhile, use a juice extractor to process the carrot, capsicum and lime. Transfer to a small jug. Squeeze all the liquid from the tea bag. Pour the tea into the jug. Add the ice cubes and stir to combine. Pour among glasses to serve.

NUTRITION VALUE

265 KJ Energy, 0.5g fat,
6g fiber, 3g protein, 12g carbs.

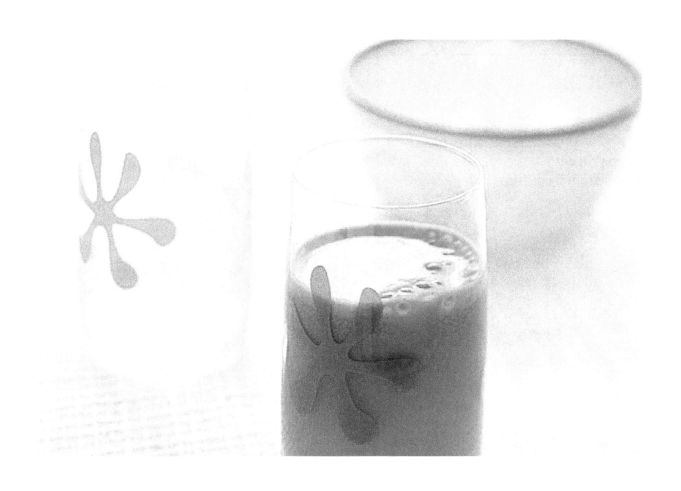

COCONUT BUTTER

Coconut butter, a creamy, tasty, and delightful recipe It's extremely easy to make and it only requires 1 ingredient and 2 minutes of your time!

MAKES 1 SERVING/ TOTAL TIME 2 MINUTE

INGREDIENTS

3 cups shredded or desiccated unsweetened coconut (270 g)

METHOD

STEP 1

Add the shredded coconut to a blender or food processor and blend until smooth.

STEP 2

Serve with some raspberry jam toasts, in smoothies like a mango smoothie, or add it to your morning oatmeal. It would also taste great on some baked sweet potatoes or squash or as a replacement for cashew butter (or any other kind of vegan butter) in any recipe.

Keep the leftovers in an airtight container in the fridge for at least 2 weeks.

| NUTRITION VALUE | 60 KJ Energy, 5.6g fat, 5g saturated fat, 1.5g fiber, 0.6g protein, 2.6g carbs. |

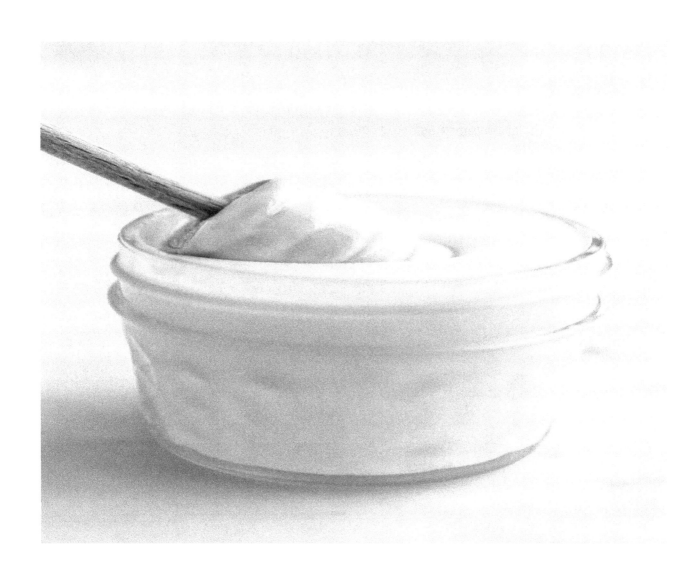

VEGAN PANCAKES

Vegan pancakes, made in less than 20 minutes with 8 simple ingredients. They're so light and fluffy, easy to make, and perfect for breakfast.

MAKES 6 SERVING/ TOTAL TIME 20 MINUTE

INGREDIENTS

1 cup whole wheat flour (120 g)

2 tbsp brown, cane or coconut sugar

2 tsp baking powder

1/4 tsp salt

3/4 cup unsweetened plant milk of your choice (190 ml), I used soy milk

1 flax egg

1 tbsp oil (optional), I used melted coconut oil

1 tsp vanilla extract (optional)

METHOD

STEP 1

Mix dry ingredients in a large bowl (flour, sugar, baking powder, and salt).

Add the liquid ingredients (milk, flax egg, oil, and vanilla extract) to the bowl and stir until well combined. Let the batter stand for 5-10 minutes before using it.

STEP 2

Place 1/4 cup of the batter (65 ml) in a lightly greased hot pan or griddle and cook for about 2 minutes for each side or until golden brown. When the underside is golden and bubbles begin to appear on the surface, it's time to flip over onto the other side.

Serve immediately with vegan butter, vegan Nutella, or even raspberry jam. You can also eat them with maple syrup, cacao nibs, and fresh fruit, or serve them with your favorite plant milk.

NUTRITION VALUE

124 KJ Energy, 3.7g fat, 2.4g saturated fat, 3.1g fiber, 3.9g protein, 20.2g carbs.

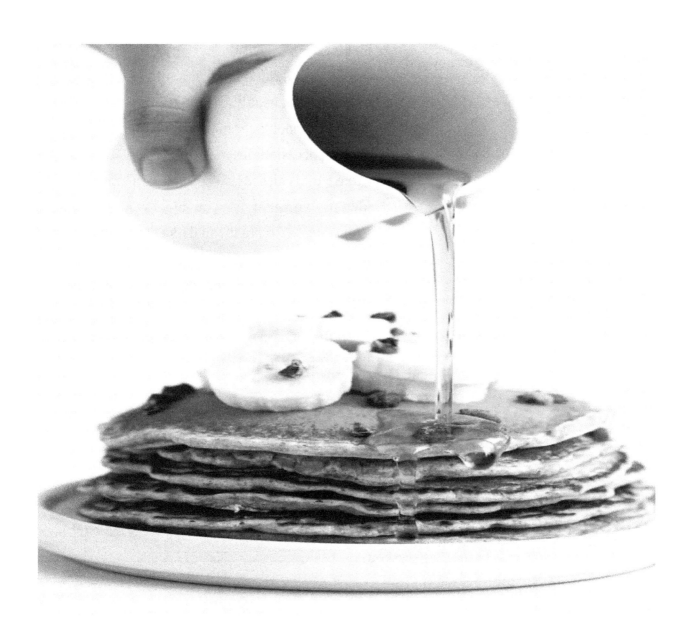

BERRY COMPOTE

Berry compote, sweet, fruity, and delicious. It's nutritious, it requires only 4 ingredients and it's ready in just 15 minutes.

MAKES 4 SERVING/ TOTAL TIME 20 MINUTE

INGREDIENTS

1 cup strawberries (150 g), chopped

1 cup blueberries (150 g)

2 tbsp orange juice

METHOD

STEP 1

Put all the ingredients together in a saucepan and cook over medium heat until it boils.

After that, cook over medium heat for 10-15 minutes, stirring occasionally.

If the fruit is already sweet, you don't need to add any kind of sweetener, but you might want to try it and add some sugar to taste if you'd like your compote sweeter.

STEP 2

Serve your favorite sweet dishes with this vegan compote for a delicious fruity taste.

Keep the leftovers in a sealed container for 7-10 days or in the freezer for up to 1 month.

NUTRITION VALUE	24 KJ Energy, 0.2g fat, 1.1g fiber, 0.4g protein, 5.9g carbs.

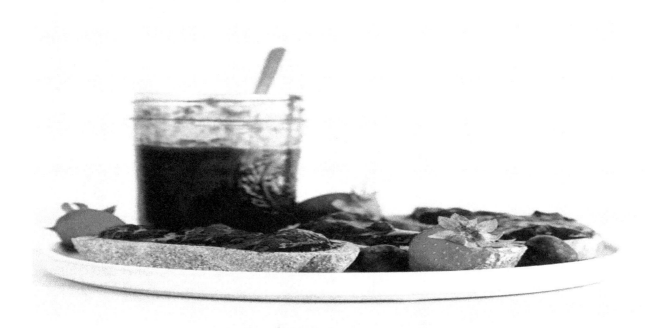

VEGAN GLUTEN FREE BLUEBERRY WAFFLES

Vegan gluten-free blueberry waffles, made with just 5 ingredients in about 30 minutes. Perfect for breakfast served with extra blueberries and maple syrup.

MAKES 5 SERVING/ TOTAL TIME 30 MINUTE

INGREDIENTS

2 and 1/2 cups rolled oats (250 g), use gluten-free if needed

1 and 1/2 cups plant milk of your choice (375 ml), we used oat milk

1/4 cup maple or agave syrup (4 tbsp)

2 tbsp flax seeds

1/2 cup fresh blueberries (80 g)

METHOD

STEP 1

Add the rolled oats to a food processor or blender and pulse until they are ground into a powder-like consistency.

Add the rest of the ingredients (except the blueberries) and pulse again until well combined.

Transfer the batter into a large mixing bowl, add the blueberries and stir until well combined.

Preheat the waffle maker according to manufacturer's directions and add some oil if needed.

Pour the batter into the waffle maker and cook according to manufacturer's instructions until golden brown. Our waffles were ready in 7 minutes.

STEP 2

Serve with your favorite toppings. We topped our waffles with extra blueberries and maple syrup.

Keep leftover waffles in a sealed container in the fridge for about 3 days or in the freezer for 1 month.

NUTRITION VALUE

205 Energy, 4.1g fat, 0.6g saturated fat, 4.7g fiber, 4.9g protein, 37g carbs.

18

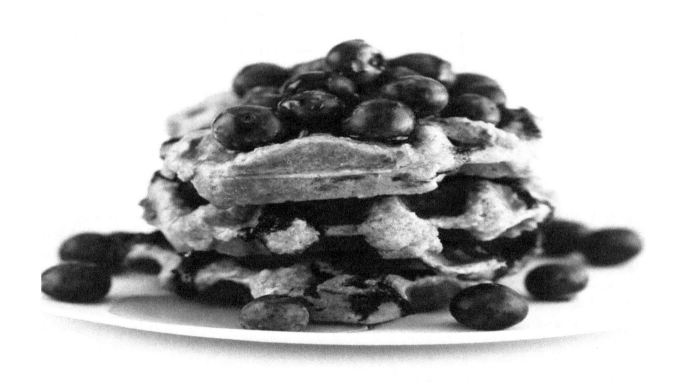

VEGAN RAWNOLA

This vegan rawnola is a raw version of granola, made with just 5 ingredients in less than 5 minutes. It's a super healthy breakfast or snack recipe!

MAKES 4 SERVING/ TOTAL TIME 5 MINUTE

INGREDIENTS

3/4 cup walnuts (90 g)

6 Medjool dates, pitted

1/2 cup oats (50 g), gluten-free if needed

2 tbsp ground flax seeds

1/2 tsp cinnamon powder

METHOD

STEP 1

Add the walnuts to a food processor and blend until they have a crumbly texture.

Add the dates and blend again.

Finally, add the rest of the ingredients and blend until well combined.

STEP 2

We served our rawnola with some banana slices and some soy milk, but you can enjoy it as is, with any plant milk, yogurt, fruit or any ingredient you want.

Keep leftovers in a sealed container at room temperature for 2 to 3 weeks or in the fridge for 3 to 4 weeks.

NUTRITION VALUE

152 KJ Energy, 7.8g fat, 0.5g saturated fat, 3.1g fiber, 4.5g protein, 18.6g carbs.

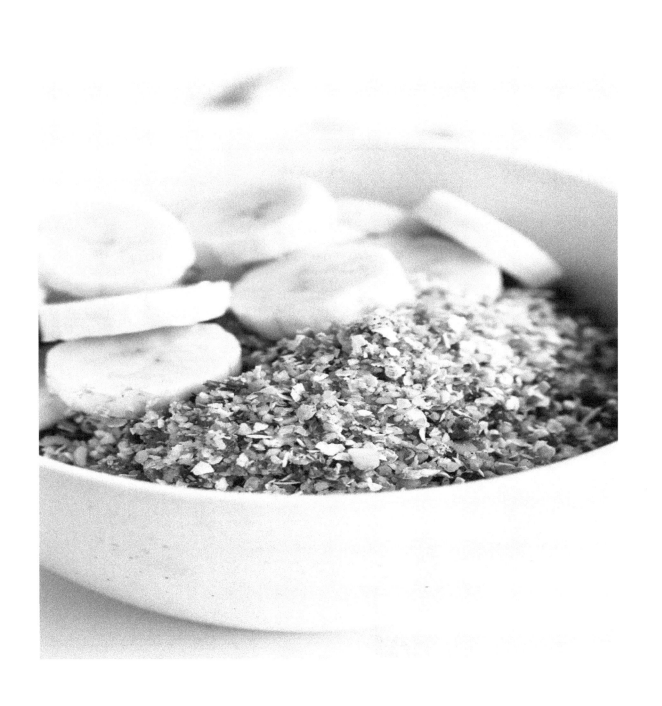

5-MINUTE OATMEAL BOWL

If you're looking for a quick, easy and super nutritious breakfast or snack recipe, this delicious oatmeal bowl is for you. It's ready in just 5 minutes!

MAKES 1 SERVING/ TOTAL TIME 5 MINUTE

INGREDIENTS

3 tbsp instant oats, use gluten-free if needed

1/4 cup or 4 tbsp boiling water

1 banana

1/2 dragon fruit, see notes

1/4 cup or 4 tbsp plant milk of your choice, we used soy milk

1 tbsp coconut yogurt

METHOD

STEP 1

Add oats and boiling water to a bowl, stir and let stand for 2 to 3 minutes. In the meanwhile, peel and chop the fruit. Add the milk, coconut yogurt and chopped fruit, stir and enjoy your oatmeal bowl.

STEP 2

We used unsweetened soy milk, but feel free to use any sweetened plant milk you want or any sweetener you have on hand.

Best when fresh, keep leftovers in a sealed container in the fridge for 1 to 2 days.

NUTRITION VALUE

254 KJ Energy, 4.8g fat, 0.4g saturated fat, 4.3g fiber, 5.8g protein, 49.9g carbs.

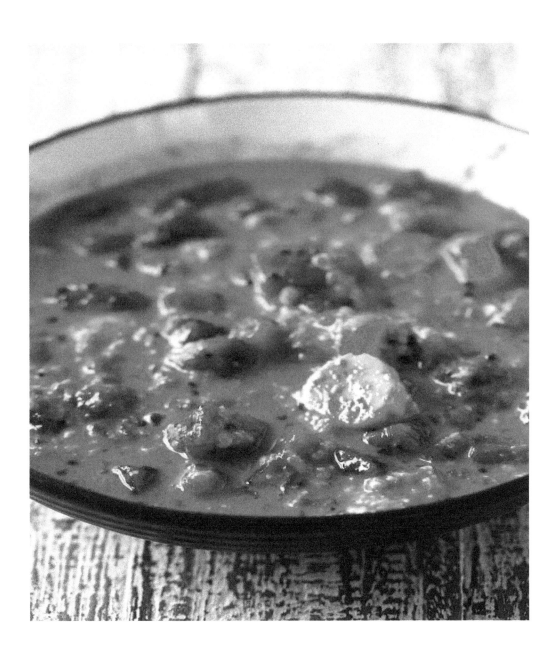

PEANUT BUTTER, BANANA, COCONUT TOAST

To make these peanut butters, banana, coconut toast you just need 4 ingredients and 10 minutes.

MAKES 1 SERVING/ TOTAL TIME 10 MINUTE

INGREDIENTS

Coconut flakes

Bread slices, see notes

Peanut or almond butter

Banana, sliced

METHOD

STEP 1

Add the coconut flakes to a skillet and cook over medium-high heat until golden brown, stirring frequently (optional).

Toast the bread slices in a skillet, toaster or oven (optional).

Spread the peanut or almond butter onto the bread slices while they're still hot (this way it will be easier and they will taste better).

Add the banana slices and top with some toasted coconut flakes.

Best with fresh, you can also eat them on the go.

NUTRITION VALUE	222 Energy, 9.7g fat, 2.5g saturated fat, 4.5g fiber, 8.3g protein, 28.4g carbs.

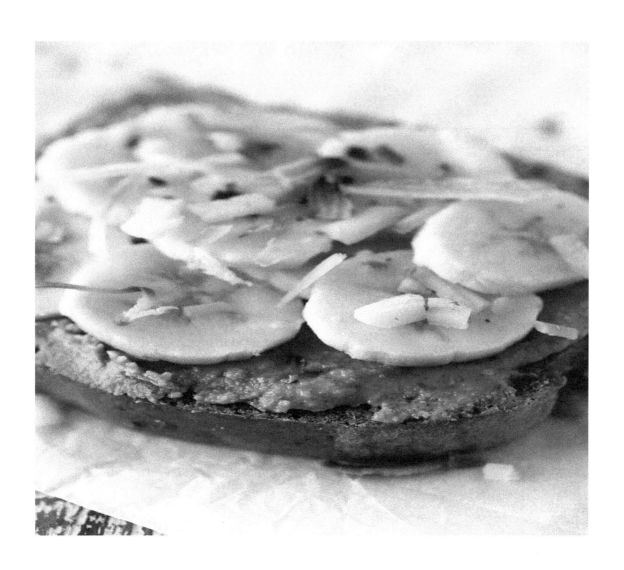

VEGAN PEANUT BUTTER AND JELLY OVERNIGHT OATS

Vegan peanut butter and jelly overnight oats, a delicious and healthy breakfast or snack to eat on the go or to make the day before to save some time every morning.

MAKES 2 SERVING/ TOTAL TIME 10 MINUTE

INGREDIENTS

3/4 cups rolled oats (90 g), gluten-free if needed

3/4 cup unsweetened soy milk (200 ml)

1 tbsp maple or agave syrup

2 tbsp peanut or almond butter

2 tbsp raspberry jam

2 bananas, chopped

Chopped peanuts (optional)

METHOD

STEP 1

There are several ways you can make this recipe. You can add all the ingredients to a jar, stir, cover and keep in the fridge overnight (or for at least 4 hours), or add all the ingredients except the bananas and add them the next morning (bananas are best when fresh and this way we prevent oxidation), or add the rolled oats and milk and add the rest of the ingredients the next morning. I prefer option number 3, but it's up to you. If you chose option number 1, you'll save some extra time every morning.

Stir the overnight oats before eating and add more milk if needed.

NUTRITION VALUE

441 Energy, 12.1g fat, 2.4g saturated fat, 7.7g fiber, 12.4g protein, 76.4g carbs.

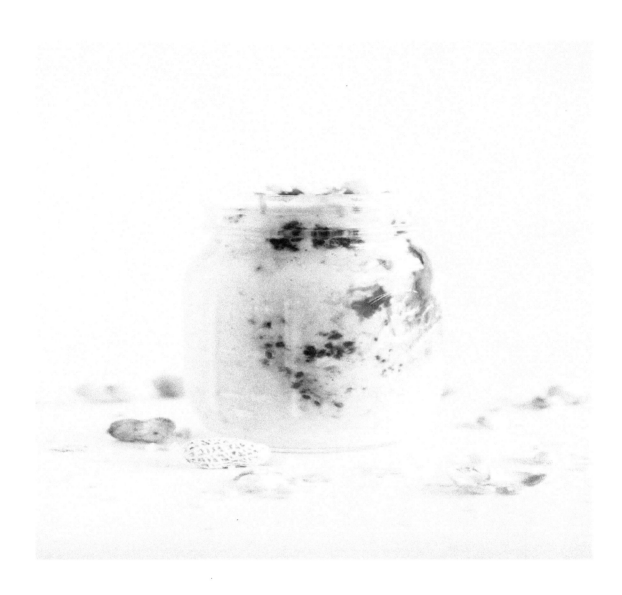

Lunch

SOUTH INDIAN BOWL

This healthy South Indian bowl packs a punch of flavor. Ready in just 30 minutes, it's a wonderful addition to your weeknight cooking repertoire.

MAKES 4 SERVING/ TOTAL TIME 30 MINUTE

INGREDIENTS

400g cauliflower florets

1 tablespoon vegetable oil

1/3 teaspoon ground turmeric

3 carrots, coarsely grated

200g green beans, trimmed, cut into 3cm pieces

1 tablespoon vegetable oil

1 teaspoon brown mustard seeds

1 red onion, finely chopped

3 sprigs fresh curry leaves

1 teaspoon cumin seeds

2 tablespoons shredded coconut

1 tablespoon lemon juice

2 x 250g pkts quinoa and brown microwave rice

100g paneer

Indian chutney, to serve

METHOD

STEP 1

Preheat oven to 200C or 180C fan-force. Line an oven tray with baking paper. Place cauliflower, vegetable oil and turmeric in a large bowl. Season and toss to coat. Arrange on prepared tray in a single layer. Roast for 25 minutes. Meanwhile, cook beans in a small saucepan of boiling salted water for 3 minutes or until tender. Drain and return to pan to keep warm.

STEP 2

Meanwhile, heat coconut oil in a large frying pan. Cook mustard seeds for 1 minute or until they start to pop. Add onion, curry leaves and cumin seeds and cook, stirring, for 5 minutes or until onion softens. Add half of onion mixture to beans. Add carrot and coconut to large pan and cook, stirring, over medium heat for 1-2 minutes

STEP 3

Divide quinoa and rice between 4 bowls. Arrange beans, carrot, cauliflower and paneer over rice. Serve with a dollop of chutney.

NUTRITION VALUE

2383 KJ Energy, 21.6g fat, 7g saturated fat, 12.2g fiber, 20.1g protein, 22g carbs.

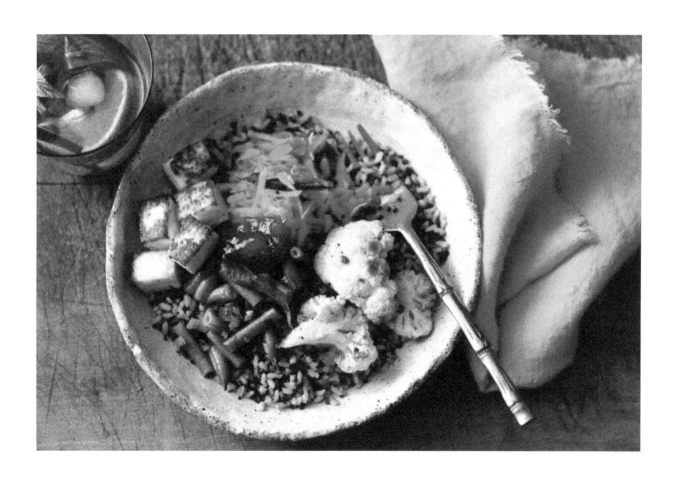

CHILLED TOFU WITH KOREAN SOY AND CHILLI DRESSING

This traditional duboo salad is a quick and delicious vegetarian side dish for your Korean banquet.

MAKES 6 SERVING/ TOTAL TIME 10 MINUTE

INGREDIENTS

300g block soft silken tofu, chilled, drained

DRESSING

1 green shallot, thinly sliced, diagonally

60ml (1/4 cup) soy sauce

1 tablespoon rice vinegar or white vinegar

1 tablespoon sesame oil

1/2 teaspoon chili powder

1 1/2 teaspoons caster sugar

1 teaspoon sesame seeds, toasted

METHOD

STEP 1

For the dressing, combine all the ingredients in a small bowl. Set aside.

STEP 2

Pat tofu dry with paper towel. Cut into 1cm-thick slices. Carefully transfer tofu to a plate. Place in the fridge until required. Pour over dressing just before serving.

NUTRITION VALUE

146 KJ Energy, 2.6g fat, 0.1g fiber, 0.8g protein, 2.1g carbs.

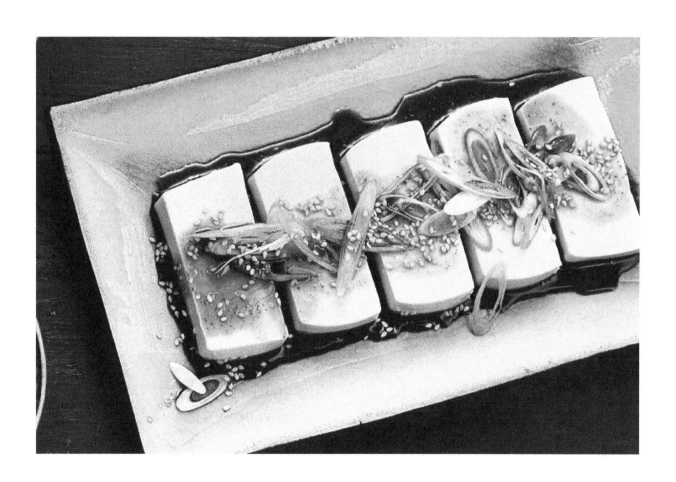

LEMON AND PISTACHIO ROASTED POTATOES

Impress your guests with these crispy golden lemon and pistachio roasted potatoes.

MAKES 8 SERVING/ TOTAL TIME 1 HOUR 10 MINUTE

INGREDIENTS

1.5kg baby cream delight potatoes

2 garlic cloves, unpeeled

1/4 cup lemon-infused extra-virgin olive oil

1/4 cup pistachio kernels, roughly chopped

Fresh flat-leaf parsley leaves, to serve

METHOD

STEP 1

Preheat oven to 200C/180C fan-forced. Line a small roasting pan with baking paper.

STEP 2

Place potatoes in a large saucepan of water over high heat. Cover. Bring to the boil. Boil for 5 minutes or until potatoes are just tender. Drain well. Transfer to prepared pan. Add garlic and 2 tablespoons oil. Toss to coat. Season with salt and pepper.

STEP 3

Roast for 45 minutes, turning potatoes halfway through, or until golden and crispy. Add pistachios to pan. Roast for a further 5 minutes.

STEP 4

Squeeze garlic from skins Discard skins. Finely chop garlic. Place in a small bowl. Add remaining oil. Whisk with a fork to combine. Drizzle over potatoes. Toss to coat. Serve sprinkled with parsley.

NUTRITION VALUE

908 KJ Energy, 9.3g fat, 1.2g saturated fat, 4.2g fiber, 5.3g protein, 25.4g carbs.

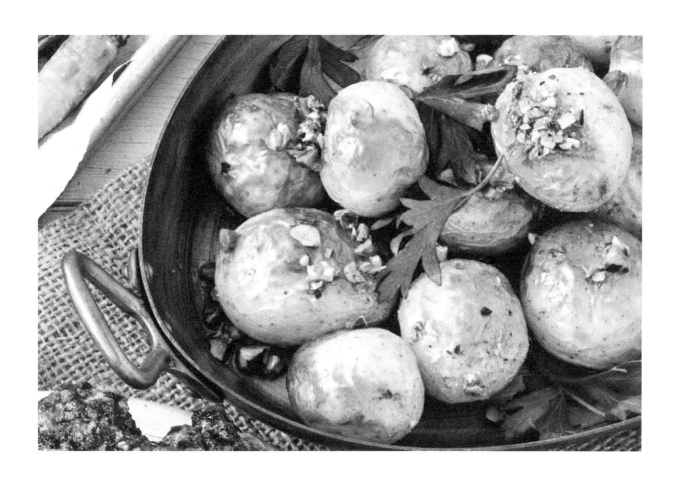

CAULIFLOWER, BROCCOLINI AND ALMOND SALAD

Good for you, versatile and super delicious, cauliflower is having a revival. Try this tasty side dish - ready in 20 minutes.

MAKES 6 SERVING/ TOTAL TIME 20 MINUTE

INGREDIENTS

600g cauliflower, cut into florets

2 bunches broccoli, trimmed, halved

1 medium carrot, cut into long matchsticks

1 long red chili, seeded, thinly sliced

2 teaspoons sesame seeds, toasted

1/4 cup natural sliced almonds, toasted

1 1/2 tablespoons kecap manis

1 1/2 tablespoons sushi seasoning

METHOD

STEP 1

Cook cauliflower in a large saucepan of boiling water for 3 minutes or until just tender. Using a slotted spoon, transfer cauliflower to a colander. Refresh under cold water. Drain well. Add broccolini to boiling water. Cook for 2 minutes or until bright green and just tender. Drain. Refresh under cold water. Drain well.

STEP 2

Place cauliflower, broccolini, carrot, chili, sesame seeds and sliced almonds in a large bowl.

STEP 3

Combine kecap manis and sushi seasoning in a jug. Drizzle over salad. Toss to combine. Season with pepper. Serve.

NUTRITION VALUE

450 KJ Energy, 2.9g fat, 0.2g saturated fat, 4g fiber, 5.9g protein, 13.2g carbs.

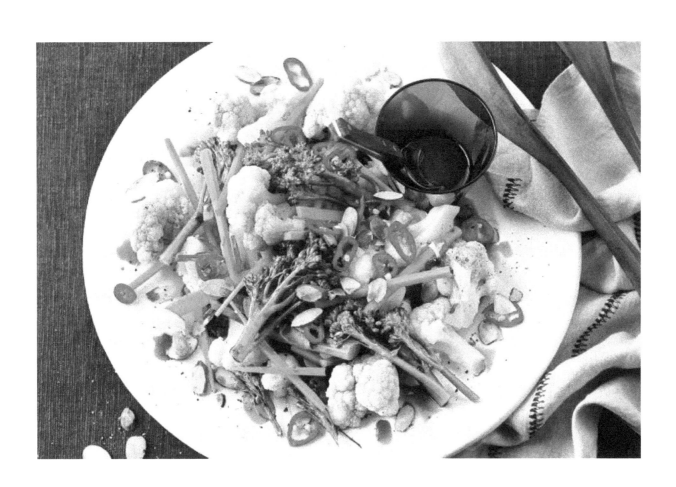

MARINATED CAULIFLOWER AND SPROUT SALAD WITH TOMATO DRESSING

For a vitamin C boost, combine cauliflower and mung bean sprouts in a salad – they're both very good sources.

MAKES 4 SERVING/ TOTAL TIME 1 HOUR 20 MINUTE

INGREDIENTS

2 tablespoons lemon juice

1 1/2 tablespoons extra-virgin olive oil

1 large tomato, finely diced

1/2 small red onion, thinly sliced

600g cauliflower, cut into small florets

1 cup mung bean sprouts, rinsed

200g snow peas, trimmed, thinly sliced

1/2 cup small fresh basil leaves

METHOD

STEP 1

Whisk lemon juice and oil in a large bowl. Add tomato, onion and cauliflower. Season with salt and pepper. Stand for 1 hour to allow flavors to develop.

STEP 2

Toss sprouts, snow peas and basil together in a serving bowl. Spoon over dressing. Serve.

NUTRITION VALUE

570 KJ Energy, 7.4g fat, 1g saturated fat, 5.6g fiber, 6.5g protein, 8g carbs.

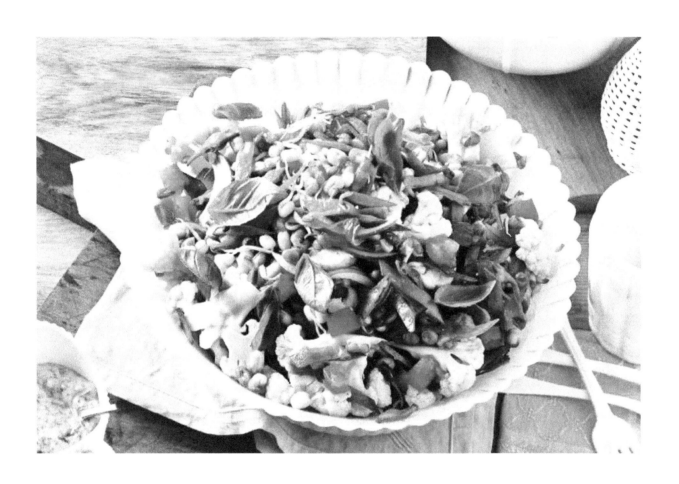

ROASTED PUMPKIN AND PARSNIP WITH SWEET GARLIC AND CRISPY SAGE

A brilliant baked pumpkin side, heart-friendly, gluten free and high in fiber.

MAKES 8 SERVING/ TOTAL TIME 45 MINUTE

INGREDIENTS

1 garlic bulb, halved crossways

1kg kent pumpkin, cut into 8 wedges (unpeeled)

4 parsnips, peeled, halved lengthways

1/4 cup extra-virgin olive oil

1 bunch fresh sage

2 tablespoons pepitas

1 tablespoon brown sugar

METHOD

STEP 1

Preheat oven to 200C/180C fan-forced. Line 2 large baking trays with baking paper.

STEP 2

Arrange garlic, pumpkin and parsnip on prepared trays. Drizzle with oil. Season with salt and pepper. Roast for 20 minutes.

STEP 3

Meanwhile, combine sage, pepitas and sugar in a bowl.

STEP 4

Sprinkle sage mixture over vegetables. Roast for 10 minutes or until golden and tender. Transfer to a platter. Serve.

NUTRITION VALUE	746 KJ Energy, 8.9g fat, 1.3g saturated fat, 5.3g fiber, 3.5g protein, 21.5g carbs.

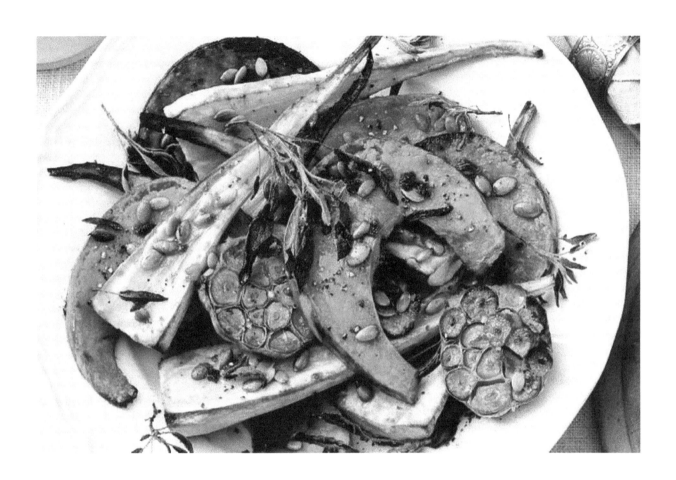

CHILLI-ROASTED PUMPKIN

Spice up roast **pumpkin** with a sprinkling of chili and crunchy pumpkin seeds.

MAKES 8 SERVING/ TOTAL TIME 45 MINUTE

INGREDIENTS

2kg butternut pumpkin, peeled, seeded, cut into 3cm pieces

1/4 cup (60ml) extra-virgin olive oil

2 tablespoons lemon juice

1 tablespoon chopped fresh rosemary

4 long red chilies, seeded, sliced

1/3 cup (80ml) extra-virgin olive oil, extra

1/3 cup (65g) pumpkin seeds (pepitas), toasted

1 tablespoon finely chopped shallot

1 tablespoon finely grated lemon zest

METHOD

STEP 1

Place a sturdy baking tray on the center rack of the oven and preheat the oven to 250°C.

STEP 2

In a large bowl, toss the pumpkin, ¼ cup (60ml) of the oil, lemon juice and rosemary. Season with salt.

STEP 3

Remove the baking tray from the oven and arrange pumpkin in an even layer over the hot tray. Roast the pumpkin, turning occasionally, for 25 mins. Add the chili and cook for a further 10 mins or until the pumpkin is caramelized and tender. Transfer to a platter.

STEP 4

Meanwhile, in a small bowl, mix the pumpkin seeds, shallot, lemon zest, and remaining 1/3 cup (80ml) oil. Drizzle over the roasted pumpkin and serve.

NUTRITION VALUE	1370KJ Energy, 21g fat, 3g saturated fat, 6g fiber, 9g protein, 23g carbs.

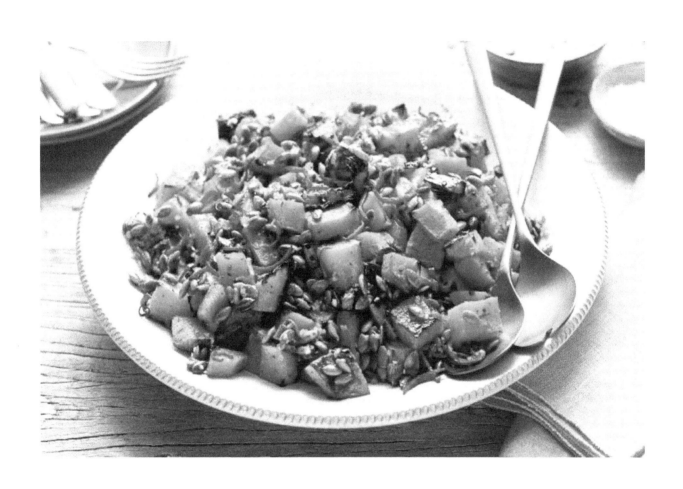

ROASTED MIXED PEAS WITH ORANGE SALT

These peas are designed to please!

MAKES 4 SERVING/ TOTAL TIME 30 MINUTE

INGREDIENTS

250g sugar snap peas, trimmed

150g snow peas, trimmed

2 garlic cloves, unpeeled

1 bunch asparagus, trimmed, halved

1/2 cup skinless hazelnuts, halved

2 tablespoons extra-virgin olive oil

ORANGE SALT

2 teaspoons orange zest

1 teaspoon sea salt

METHOD

STEP 1

Preheat oven to 220C/200C fan-forced.

STEP 2

Place peas, garlic, asparagus and hazelnuts in a roasting pan. Drizzle with 1/2 the oil. Season with pepper.

STEP 3

Roast for 20 minutes, tossing mixture halfway through cooking, until peas are just tender and lightly charred on edges.

STEP 4

Carefully squeeze garlic from skins and finely chop. Whisk garlic and remaining oil in a small bowl. Drizzle over pea mixture. Toss to coat.

STEP 5

Make Orange salt: Combine orange zest and salt in a small bowl. Sprinkle over pea mixture. Serve.

NUTRITION VALUE	1027 KJ Energy, 20.1g fat, 1.8g saturated fat, 4g fiber, 6.7g protein, 6.5g carbs.

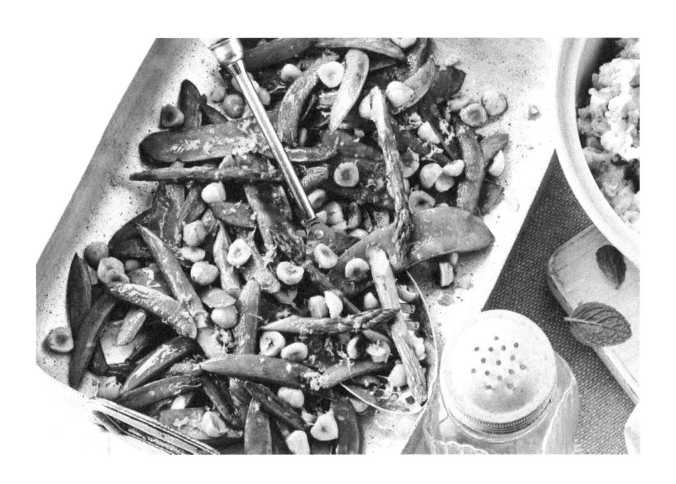

PICKLED QUKES

It's easy to make pickles at home – throw them into salads
and Asian dressings, use to top burgers, or eat 'em straight out of the jar!

MAKES 750 ML JAR SERVING/ TOTAL TIME 1 HOUR 15 MINUTE

INGREDIENTS

2 (250g) pkt Qukes (baby snacking
cucumbers), scrubbed, quartered
lengthways

1 tablespoon sea salt

160ml (2/3 cup) white wine vinegar

160ml (2/3 cup) water

1 teaspoon coriander seeds

1/2 teaspoon black peppercorns

4 whole cloves

2 fresh bay leaves

2 sprigs fresh tarragon

METHOD

STEP 1

Combine the Qukes and salt in a bowl. Toss to combine.
Cover with plastic wrap. Set aside for 1 hour to allow
water to be drawn out. Rinse. Pat dry with paper towel.

STEP 2

Combine the vinegar and water in a saucepan. Bring to
a simmer over medium heat. Simmer for 2 minutes.

STEP 3

Pack the Qukes, coriander seeds, peppercorns, cloves,
bay leaves and tarragon in a sterilized 750ml jar. Pour
over the hot vinegar mixture to cover. Seal and set aside
for 1 week before eating. Serve pickles with pate, a
terrine or cheese.

NUTRITION VALUE

46 KJ Energy, 0.1g fat,
0.1g fiber, 0.3g protein, 2g carbs.

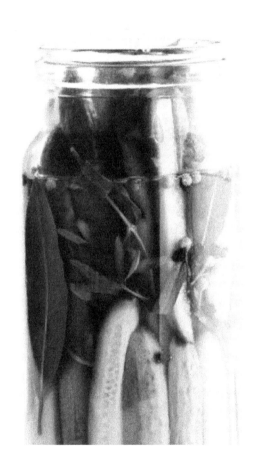

MISO, TOFU & NOODLE SOUP

The vegetables are the heroes of this Japanese-style soup.

MAKES 4 SERVING/ TOTAL TIME 15 MINUTE

INGREDIENTS

1.5L (6 cups) boiling water

2 tablespoons miso paste

2 x 190g pkts udon noodles

2 carrots, peeled, cut into matchsticks

2 green shallots, ends trimmed, cut into 5cm lengths, thinly sliced lengthways

1 bunch asparagus, woody ends trimmed, thinly sliced diagonally

300g silken tofu, cut into 2cm pieces

1/4 cup finely chopped fresh chives

METHOD

STEP 1

Place the water in a large saucepan over medium heat. Add the miso and stir to combine. Reduce heat to low. Add the noodles and gently stir to separate. Add the carrot, shallot and asparagus and cook for 1 minute or until asparagus is bright green and tender crisp.

STEP 2

Divide the noodles and soup among serving bowls. Top with tofu and sprinkle with chives. Serve immediately.

NUTRITION VALUE

946 KJ Energy, 3g fat, 1g saturated fat, 5g fiber, 14g protein, 32g carbs.

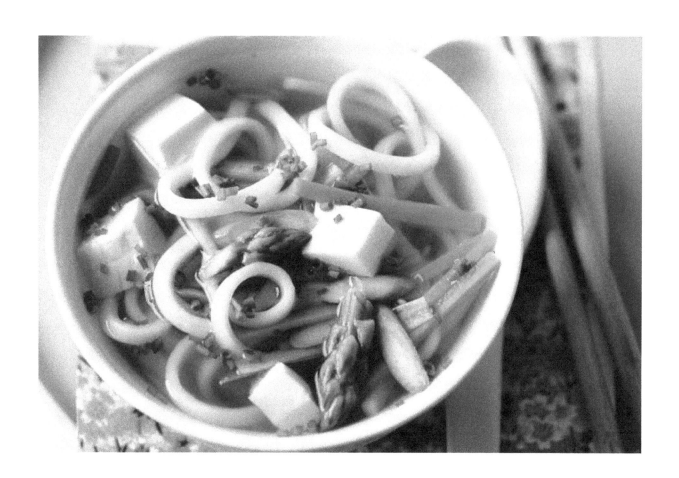

Dinner

SAUTEED POTATOES IN GARLIC OIL

Spend that extra time with this recipe and create crispy golden potato bites that will spectacularly complement any roast dinner.

MAKES 8 SERVING/ TOTAL TIME 1 HOUR 20 MINUTE

INGREDIENTS

150ml peanut oil

8 large garlic cloves, peeled, thinly sliced

1kg Sebago potatoes, peeled, cut into 3-4cm pieces

Handful fresh sage leaves

METHOD

STEP 1

Heat the oil in a small saucepan over very low heat until shimmering. Add the garlic. Cook, over a very low heat, for 20 minutes or until golden and crisp but not burnt. Use a slotted spoon to transfer the garlic to a plate lined with paper towel to drain. Strain the oil through a fine sieve into a jug, repeating to remove all sediment.

STEP 2

Boil the potato in a saucepan of lightly salted boiling water for 12-15 minutes or until just tender. Drain. Refresh under cold running water. Set aside to cool and dry. Heat 80ml (1/3 cup) of the garlic oil in a large frying pan over medium heat. Cook the potato, in 2 batches, stirring frequently, for 10-15 minutes or until crisp and golden. Use a slotted spoon to transfer to a warmed plate.

STEP 3

Wipe the pan clean with paper towel. Add a little more oil to the pan over high heat and fry the sage leaves for a few seconds until crisp. Stir in the garlic and drizzle over the potato. Season.

NUTRITION VALUE	1190 KJ Energy, 8.7g fat, 1.9g saturated fat, 13.6g fiber, 11.3g protein, 32.2g carbs.

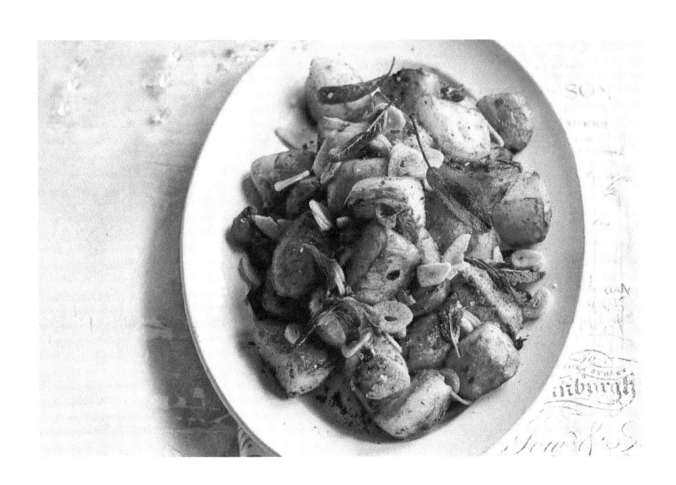

SPICY BLACK BEAN AND CORN SOUP WITH CHILLI

This spicy, satisfying **vegetarian** soup has a creamy texture and is rich in protein and fiber, thanks to the black beans.

MAKES 4 SERVING/ TOTAL TIME 8 HOUR 30 MINUTE

INGREDIENTS

220g (1 cup) dried black beans, rinsed, drained

2 teaspoons extra-virgin olive oil

1 large brown onion, finely chopped

2 celery sticks, finely chopped

2 garlic cloves, crushed

2 teaspoons ground cumin

2 teaspoons sweet paprika

1/2 teaspoon chili flakes

400g can crushed tomatoes

1.25L (5 cups) water

300g sweet potato, peeled, chopped

1 large sweet corn cob, kernels removed

2 tablespoons fresh coriander leaves, chopped

1 long fresh green chili, deseeded, finely chopped

METHOD

STEP 1

Place black beans in a large saucepan. Cover with enough cold water to come 5cm above beans. Bring to the boil over medium high heat. Cook for 10 minutes. Drain well.

STEP 2

Meanwhile, heat oil in a large non-stick frying pan over medium heat. Cook onion and celery, stirring, for 5 minutes or until soft. Add garlic, cumin, paprika and chili. Cook, stirring, for 1 minute or until aromatic.

STEP 3

Place onion mixture, beans, tomato and water in a large (6L) slow cooker. Cover. Cook on low for 7 hours. Add sweet potato and corn. Cover. Cook for a further 1 hour or until potato is tender and soup is thick. Season.

STEP 4

Combine coriander and green chili in a bowl. Divide soup among bowls. Top with coriander mixture. Serve with lime.

NUTRITION VALUE

1453 KJ Energy, 14g fat, 2g saturated fat, 17g fiber, 21g protein, 29g carbs.

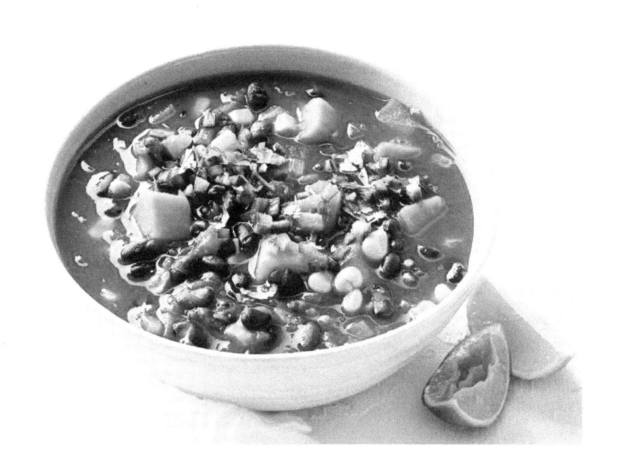

AYURVEDIC BEETROOT CURRY

Increase your vitality and health and tuck into this tasty curry tonight!

MAKES 4 SERVING/ TOTAL TIME 1 HOUR 50 MINUTE

INGREDIENTS

1.5kg beetroot, peeled, cut into 3cm cubes

2 tablespoons fresh ginger, grated

3 garlic cloves, crushed

2 teaspoons garam masala

2 teaspoons ground cumin

1 teaspoon ground coriander

1 teaspoon ground turmeric

400g can coconut cream

2 tablespoons coconut oil

2 brown onions, thinly sliced

4 sprigs fresh curry leaves

400g can chickpeas, drained, rinsed

1/3 cup red lentils, rinsed, drained

100g baby spinach

1 tablespoon lemon juice

Sprigs coriander, to serve

METHOD

STEP 1

Combine beetroot, ginger, garlic, spices and coconut cream in a large bowl. Toss to coat.

STEP 2

Heat coconut oil in a large saucepan over high heat. Cook onion and curry leaves, stirring, for 5 minutes or until well browned. Add beetroot mixture, chickpeas, lentils and 1 cup water. Season and stir to combine. Bring to the boil. Reduce heat to low and cook, covered, for 1 hour 15 minutes or until lentils and beetroot are tender. Stir in spinach and lemon juice. Serve sprinkled with coriander.

NUTRITION VALUE

2696 KJ Energy, 32.9g fat, 27.3g saturated fat, 21.6g fiber, 19.3g protein, 76.4g carbs.

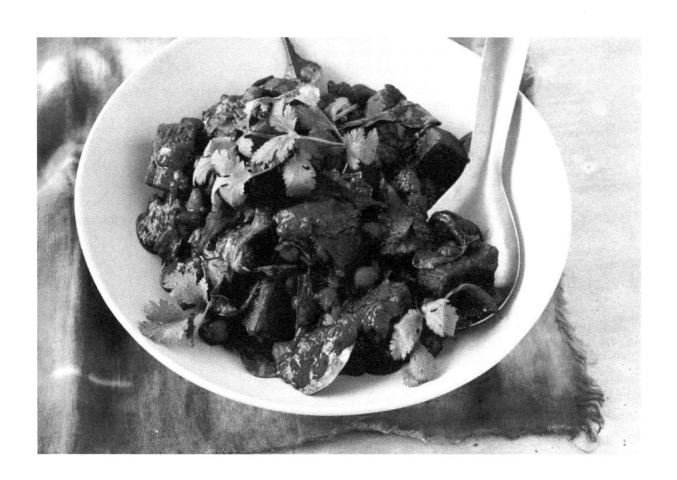

LENTIL, SPINACH & TOMATO SALAD

Recipe that everyone loves!

MAKES 4 SERVING/ TOTAL TIME 15 MINUTE

INGREDIENTS

2 x 400g cans brown lentils, rinsed, drained

4 ripe tomatoes, coarsely chopped

80g baby spinach leaves

100g flat beans, topped, cut into 2cm lengths diagonally

2 carrots, peeled, coarsely chopped

2 Lebanese cucumbers, coarsely chopped

1/2 cup chopped fresh continental parsley

1 tablespoon fresh lemon juice

1 tablespoon balsamic vinegar

1 tablespoon extra-virgin olive oil

1 garlic clove, crushed

Sliced crusty bread, to serve

METHOD
STEP 1
Place the lentils, tomato, spinach, beans, carrot, cucumber and parsley in a large bowl and gently toss until just combined.

STEP 2
Use a balloon whisk to whisk together the lemon juice, vinegar, oil and garlic in a small bowl. Season with pepper.

STEP 3
Drizzle the dressing over the salad and toss until well combined. Divide the salad among serving bowls. Serve with crusty bread.

NUTRITION VALUE

800 KJ Energy, 5g fat, 1g saturated fat, 10g fiber, 12g protein, 19g carbs.

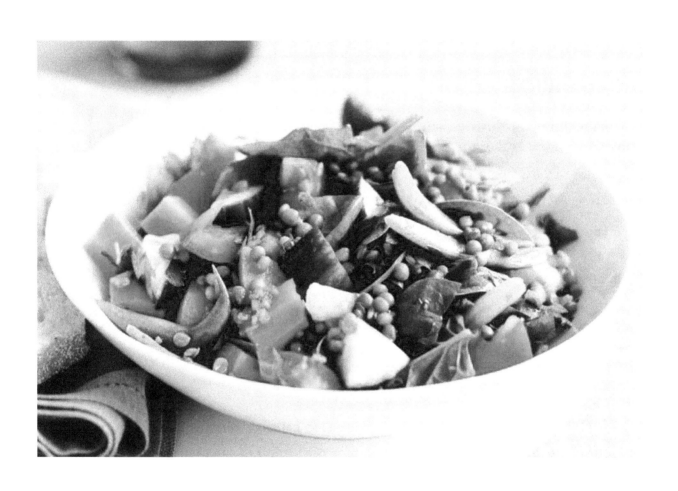

BROWN RICE AND HARISSA ROASTED VEGETABLE SALAD

This colorful salad incorporates all our favorite roast vegetables with tasty brown rice and spicy harissa.

MAKES 4 SERVING/ TOTAL TIME 45 MINUTE

INGREDIENTS

1 cup medium-grain brown rice, rinsed

1 medium red capsicum, chopped

1 medium yellow capsicum, chopped

1/2 small orange sweet potato, thinly sliced

2 small zucchinis, halved, chopped

2 baby eggplant, halved, chopped

1 tablespoon harissa

1/4 cup extra-virgin olive oil

2 teaspoons finely grated lemon rind

2 tablespoons lemon juice

1 tablespoon chopped fresh oregano leaves

fresh oregano leaves, to serve

METHOD

STEP 1

Preheat oven to 220°C/ 200°C fan-forced. Cook rice in a large saucepan of boiling, salted water, following packet directions, until tender. Drain.

STEP 2

Meanwhile, place capsicum, potato, zucchinis, eggplant, harissa and 1 tablespoon oil in a roasting pan. Toss to combine. Roast for 20 minutes or until vegetables are tender.

STEP 3

Place rice, capsicum mixture, remaining oil, lemon rind, lemon juice and oregano in a large bowl. Season with salt and pepper. Toss to combine. Top with oregano leaves. Serve.

NUTRITION VALUE

1439 KJ Energy, 16g fat, 3g saturated fat, 4g fiber, 5g protein, 44g carbs.

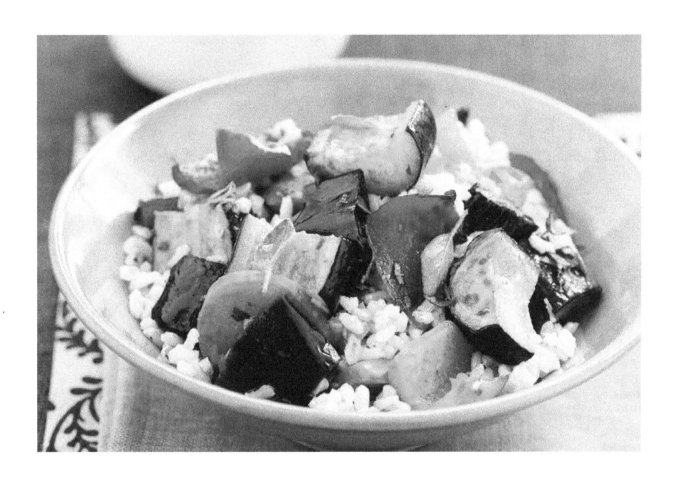

ORANGE SALAD

Make the most of oranges at the peak of their season in this sensational salad.

MAKES 6 SERVING/ TOTAL TIME 10 MINUTE

INGREDIENTS

4 large oranges, peeled, pith removed and discarded, sliced into 2cm rounds

1 red onion, finely sliced

3 tablespoons finely chopped flat-leaf parsley

1/4 cup (60ml) olive oil

1 tablespoon orange juice

2 teaspoons orange blossom water*

2 tablespoons slivered pistachios, to serve

METHOD
STEP 1

Lay oranges on a platter. Sprinkle with onion and parsley. Combine oil, juice and blossom water and season. Dress salad just before serving and season with freshly ground pepper. Garnish with nuts.

NUTRITION VALUE

516 KJ Energy, 8g fat, 1g saturated fat, 3g fiber, 2g protein, 9g carbs.

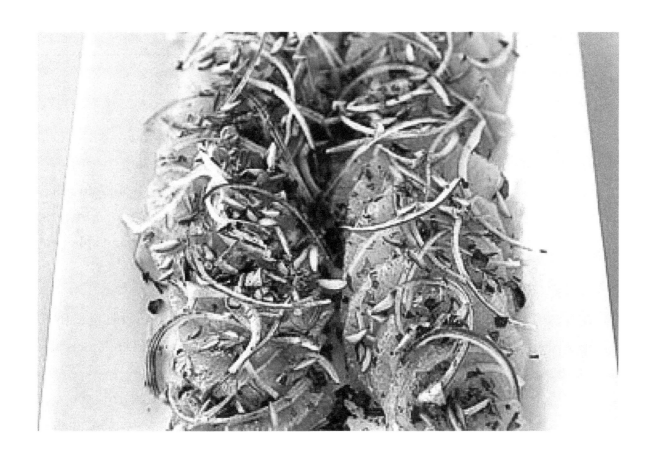

MOROCCAN PUMPKIN SOUP

Take an Australian classic like pumpkin soup, add a Moroccan twist and make this "souper" meal which is vegan friendly.

MAKES 6 SERVING/ TOTAL TIME 1 HOUR 25 MINUTE

INGREDIENTS

1/4 cup (60ml) olive oil

1 leek, white part only, thinly sliced

3 cloves garlic, finely chopped

1 red birdseye chili, finely chopped

1 cinnamon stick

3cm piece ginger, peeled, thinly sliced

1 1/2 teaspoons cumin seeds

2 carrots, peeled, coarsely chopped

1.5kg butternut or Queensland blue pumpkin, peeled, seeded cut into 3cm pieces

1/3 cup (70g) yellow split peas

Juice of 1/2 lemon

Coriander sprigs, to serve

Soup sprinkles, to serve

METHOD

STEP 1

Heat oil in a large saucepan over low-medium heat and cook leek, garlic and 2 teaspoons salt, stirring occasionally, for 3 minutes or until soft. Add chili, cinnamon, ginger and cumin and stir for 1 minute or until fragrant. Add carrots, pumpkin and split peas. Stir to coat in onion mixture.

STEP 2

Add 1.5 liters water to saucepan and bring to the boil, then simmer for 50 minutes or until split peas are soft.

STEP 3

Remove and discard cinnamon stick from soup. Add lemon juice then process or blend soup, in small batches, in a food processor or blender until smooth. Return soup to pan and reheat over medium heat. Serve topped with coriander sprigs and soup sprinkles.

NUTRITION VALUE

1066 KJ Energy, 11g fat, 2g saturated fat, 8g fiber, 9g protein, 26g carbs.

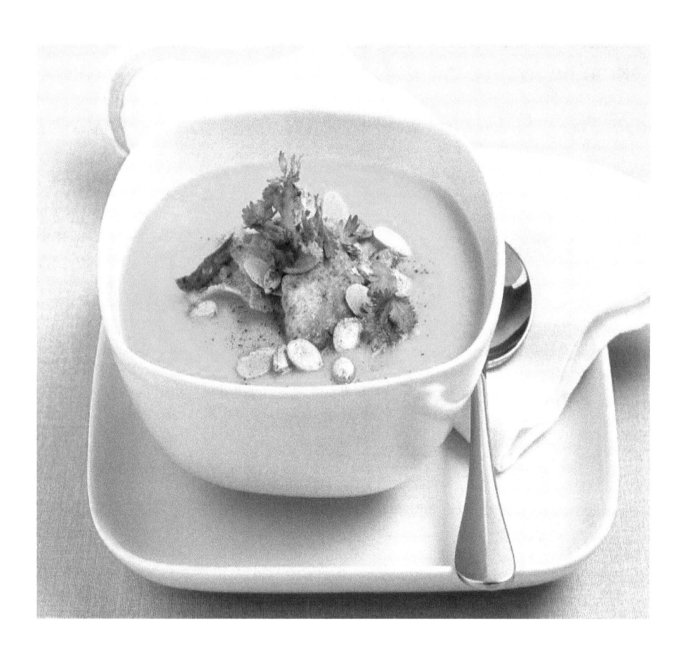

LENTIL SOUP

This old favorite is best served with chunks of crusty bread to mop up every last skerrick.

MAKES 4 SERVING/ TOTAL TIME 35 MINUTE

INGREDIENTS

1 tablespoon olive oil

1 brown onion, finely chopped

1 carrot, peeled, finely chopped

1 celery stick, trimmed, finely chopped

2 x 400g cans brown lentils, rinsed, drained

400g can diced tomatoes

500ml (2 cups) Massel vegetable liquid stock

2 dried bay leaves

2 teaspoons dried oregano leaves

1/4 cup chopped fresh continental parsley

Olive oil (optional), to drizzle

25g (1/3 cup) finely grated parmesan

METHOD

STEP 1

Heat the oil in a large saucepan over medium heat. Cook onion, carrot and celery, stirring occasionally, for 5 minutes or until soft. Stir in lentils, tomato, stock, bay leaves and oregano. Reduce heat to low. Simmer for 10 minutes or until mixture reduces slightly. Set aside for 5 minutes to cool. Remove and discard the bay leaves.

STEP 2

Process half the soup in a food processor until smooth. Return to the pan. Cook, stirring, over medium heat until heated through. Stir in the parsley.

STEP 3

Divide among serving bowls. Drizzle over oil, if desired. Top with parmesan.

NUTRITION VALUE	867 KJ Energy, 8g fat, 2g saturated fat, 8g fiber, 13g protein, 17g carbs.

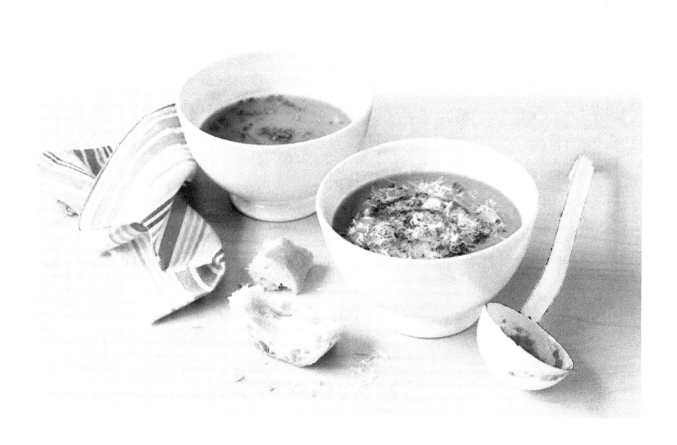

SPINACH DHAL WITH GARLIC BREAD

A satisfying **vegan** meal of tasty lentils served with warm and delicious garlic bread.

MAKES 4 SERVING/ TOTAL TIME 30 MINUTE

INGREDIENTS

1 tablespoon olive oil

1 brown onion, halved, finely chopped

8 baby desiree potatoes, quartered

1 teaspoon ground cumin

1 teaspoon ground coriander

500ml (2 cups) water

1 tablespoon tomato paste

1 x 400g can brown lentils, rinsed, drained

80g baby spinach leaves

GARLIC BREAD

2 pieces (22cm-diameter) Lebanese bread

1 tablespoon olive oil

2 garlic cloves, crushed

METHOD

STEP 1

Preheat oven to 180°C. Heat the oil in a saucepan over medium heat. Add the onion and potato and cook, stirring, for 5 minutes or until the onion is soft. Add the cumin and coriander and cook, stirring, for 1 minute or until aromatic.

STEP 2

Add the water and tomato paste and bring to the boil. Reduce heat to medium and simmer, stirring occasionally, for 10 minutes or until liquid reduces by half.

STEP 3

Meanwhile, to make the garlic bread, place the bread on a baking tray. Combine the oil and garlic in a small bowl. Brush both sides of the bread evenly with garlic mixture. Season with salt. Bake for 8 minutes or until crisp. Break into wedges.

STEP 4

Add the lentils to the potato mixture and cook for 2 minutes or until heated through. Add spinach and stir until just wilted. Season with salt and pepper.

NUTRITION VALUE

1585 KJ Energy, 8g fat, 1g saturated fat, 9g fiber, 14g protein, 63g carbs.

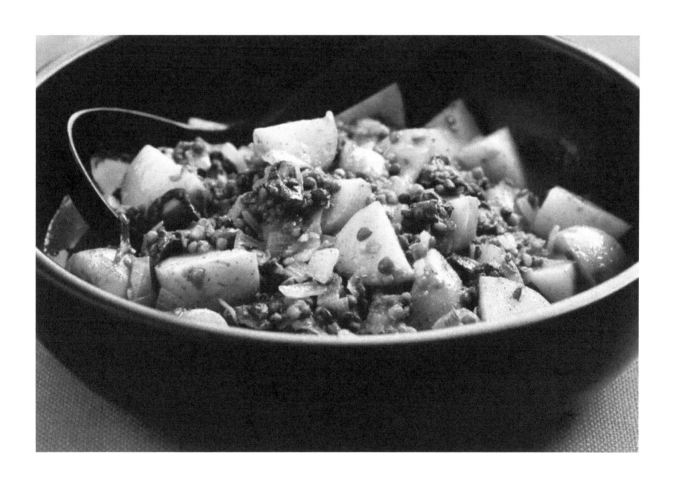

ASIAN-STYLE CURRIED VEGETABLE BROTH

Create a richly flavorsome curry soup using tofu, rice noodles and a handful of fresh ingredients.

MAKES 4 SERVING/ TOTAL TIME 30 MINUTE

INGREDIENTS

1/4 cup green curry paste

320g packet nigari tofu (extra firm), cut into 2cm cubes

150ml light coconut milk

2 cups Massel vegetable liquid stock

2 1/2 cups water

80g dried rice vermicelli noodles

1 bunch gai plum, stalks diagonally sliced, leaves shredded

125g packet fresh baby corn, halved lengthways

Coriander leaves, to serve

METHOD

STEP 1

Heat curries paste in a large wok over medium heat, stirring, for 1 to 2 minutes, or until aromatic. Add tofu. Cook, tossing gently, for 1 minute. Add coconut milk, stock and water. Bring to a simmer.

STEP 2

Add noodles and gai lum stalks to wok. Cook for 5 minutes, or until noodles are almost tender.

STEP 3

Add gai lum leaves and corn to wok. Cook for 2 to 3 minutes, or until leaves wilt. Divide broth between 4 serving bowls. Top with coriander. Serve.

NUTRITION VALUE

100KJ Energy, 13.6g fat, 2.5g saturated fat, 6g fiber, 14.6g protein, 23.8g carbs.

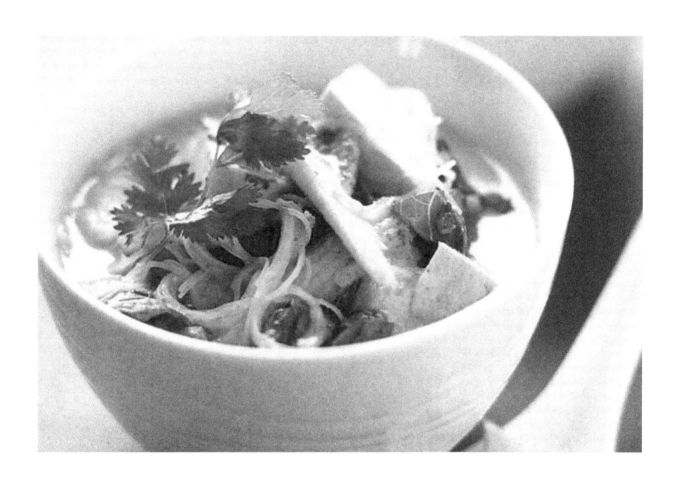

Snacks

LENTIL BURGERS WITH TAHINI SAUCE

Spicy lentil burgers topped with avocado and tahini sauce will have everyone asking for more.

MAKES 4 SERVING/ TOTAL TIME 35 MINUTE

INGREDIENTS

1 teaspoon olive oil

1 onion, finely chopped

1 garlic clove, crushed

1 teaspoon ground cumin

2 cups cooked brown lentils

1/2 cup (35g) fresh wholemeal breadcrumbs

2 teaspoons soy sauce

Salt & freshly ground pepper

4 wholemeal bread rolls, halved

1 small avocado

Mixed salad leaves

2 medium beetroot bulbs, peeled, coarsely grated

2 carrots, peeled, coarsely grated

SAUCE

1/3 cup (95g) tahini

2 tablespoons fresh lemon juice

1 garlic clove, crushed

METHOD

STEP 1

Preheat oven to 180°C. Line a baking tray with non-stick paper. Heat oil in a pan over medium heat. Cook onion and garlic for 3 mins until soft. Add cumin, cook for 30 secs. Remove from heat.

STEP 2

Place onion mixture, cooked lentils, breadcrumbs and soy sauce in a bowl. Season. Use clean hands to combine, mushing the lentils slightly so they will bind. Divide into four portions. Shape into patties. Place on tray. Cook for 30 mins, turns halfway through cooking.

STEP 3

Meanwhile, combine tahini, lemon juice, garlic and 2 tablespoons water until smooth.

STEP 4

Toast rolls then spread with avocado. Top with mixed leaves, grated beetroot and carrot, lentil burger, some tahini sauce and the bun lid.

NUTRITION VALUE

2507 KJ Energy, 28g fat, 5g saturated fat, 23g protein, 54g carbs.

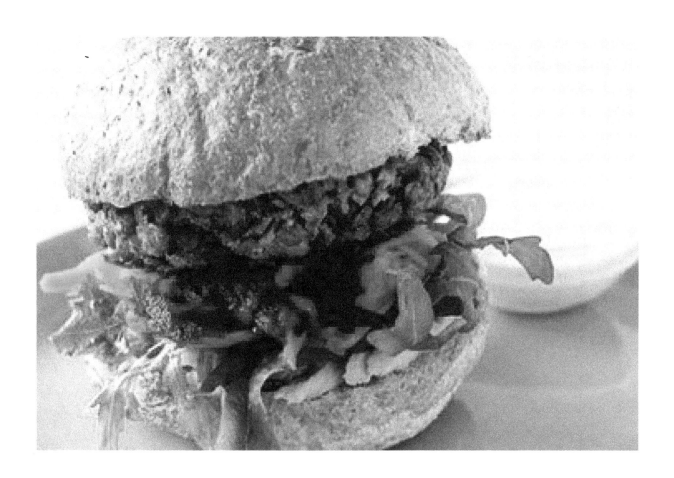

MOROCCAN HOMMUS DIP

A little Moroccan seasoning lifts the flavor of homemade hummus.

MAKES 8 SERVING / TOTAL TIME 10 MINUTE

INGREDIENTS

2 x 400g cans chickpeas, drained, rinsed

2 lemons, juiced

2 1/2 tablespoons extra-virgin olive oil

2 garlic cloves, crushed

1 1/2 teaspoons Moroccan seasoning mix

1 teaspoon cracked black pepper

1 tablespoon flat-leaf parsley leaves, roughly chopped

METHOD

STEP 1

1 Place chickpeas, 1/2 cup lemon juice, 2 tablespoons oil, garlic, Moroccan seasoning and pepper in a food processor. Process until smooth. Transfer to an airtight container. Cover and refrigerate until ready to serve.

STEP 2

2 Spoon dip into a serving bowl. Sprinkle with parsley and pepper. Drizzle with remaining oil. Serve.

NUTRITION VALUE	516 KJ Energy, 7g fat, 1g saturated fat, 4g protein, 9g carbs.

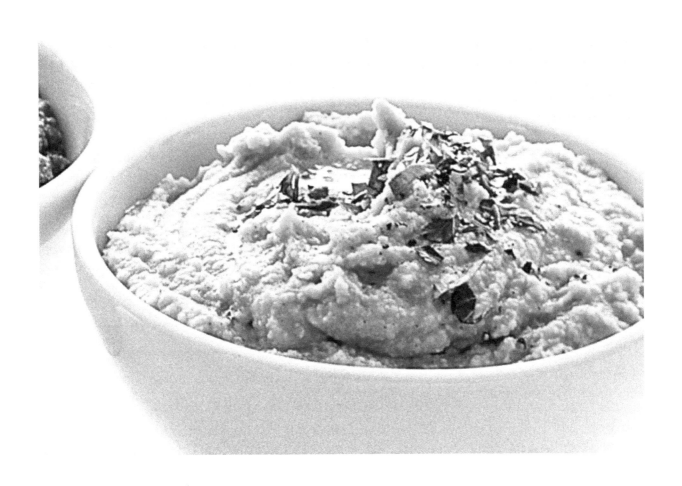

ROASTED TOMATO SOUP WITH TOAST STARS

Kids will just love this delicious roast tomato soup with fun toast stars which is also **vegan** friendly.

MAKES 6 SERVING/ TOTAL TIME 50 MINUTE

INGREDIENTS

1/4 cup (60ml) olive oil

1 onion, finely chopped

1kg vine-ripened tomatoes, roughly chopped

3 garlic cloves

1 teaspoon caster sugar

600ml Massel vegetable liquid stock

100g alphabet pasta or risoni

2 slices bread, toasted

METHOD

STEP 1

Preheat the oven to 200C.

STEP 2

Heat oil in a shallow ovenproof casserole; add onion and cook over low heat, stirring occasionally, for about 10 minutes or until softened. Add tomatoes, garlic, and sugar, and season well with salt and pepper. Roast uncovered in oven for 20 minutes, then allow mixture to cool. Puree in a blender, adding a little of the stock if the mixture is too thick. Return to pan and add remaining stock. Bring to the boil, add pasta and simmer for 10 minutes. Taste and adjust seasoning if necessary. Cut stars from toast slices with a star cutter, and serve with soup.

NUTRITION VALUE

880 KJ Energy, 8g fat, 2g saturated fat, 6g protein, 22g carbs.

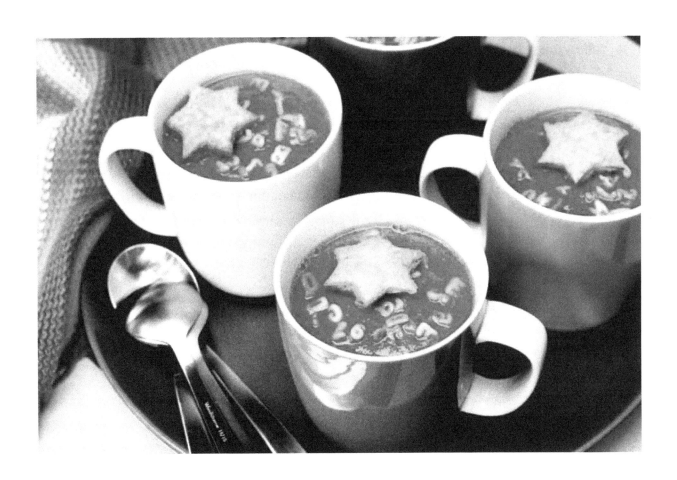

GARLICKY SQUASH

This recipe is vegan friendly.

MAKES 12 SERVING/ TOTAL TIME 15 MINUTE

INGREDIENTS

1kg yellow squash, halved

1 tablespoon extra-virgin olive oil

3 garlic cloves, crushed

4 green shallots, ends trimmed, thinly sliced

METHOD

STEP 1

Cook the squash in a large saucepan of boiling water for 4-5 minutes or until just tender. Drain well.

STEP 2

Heat the oil in a large frying pan over medium heat. Add garlic and cook for 30 seconds or until aromatic. Add the squash and cook, stirring, for 2 minutes or until heated through. Add the shallot and cook, stirring, for 1 minute or until combined. Transfer to a bowl to serve.

NUTRITION VALUE	166 KJ Energy, 2g fat, 2g protein, 2g carbs.

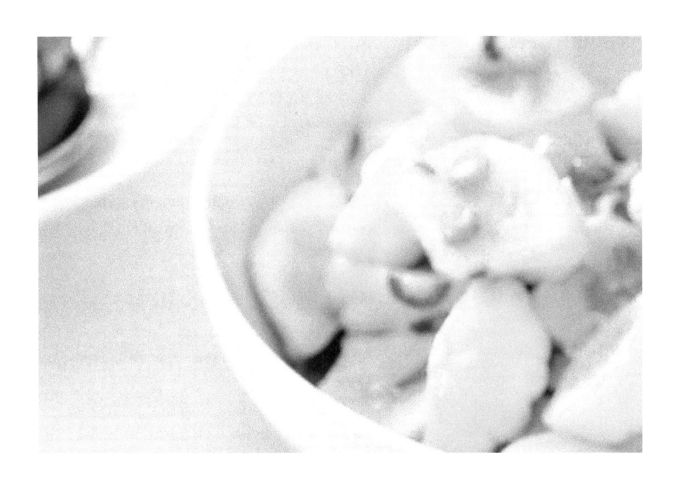

ROAST CAPSICUM & CHICKPEA DIP

Recipe that everyone loves!

MAKES 10 SERVING/ TOTAL TIME 30 MINUTE

INGREDIENTS

1 red capsicum quartered

1 long red chili

1/3 cup (80ml) olive oil, plus extra to drizzle

420g can chickpeas, rinsed, drained

2 tablespoons tahini

1 garlic clove

1/4 cup (60ml) lemon juice

1/4 cup coriander leaves, plus extra to garnish

Corn chips*, to serve

Chili oil* (optional), to serve

METHOD

STEP 1

Heat the grill to high. Place the capsicum skin-side up on a baking tray with the chili and drizzle with extra olive oil.

STEP 2

Grill for 3-4 minutes until skins are charred. Place in a plastic bag, seal and leave to sweat for 15 minutes, then peel.

STEP 3

Place capsicum and chili flesh in a food processor with olive oil, chickpeas, tahini, garlic, lemon juice and coriander. Process to a smooth paste and season.

STEP 4

Transfer to a serving bowl, garnish with extra coriander, and drizzle with chili oil if desired. Serve with corn chips.

NUTRITION VALUE	521 KJ Energy, 10g fat, 2g saturated fat, 3g protein, 5g carbs.

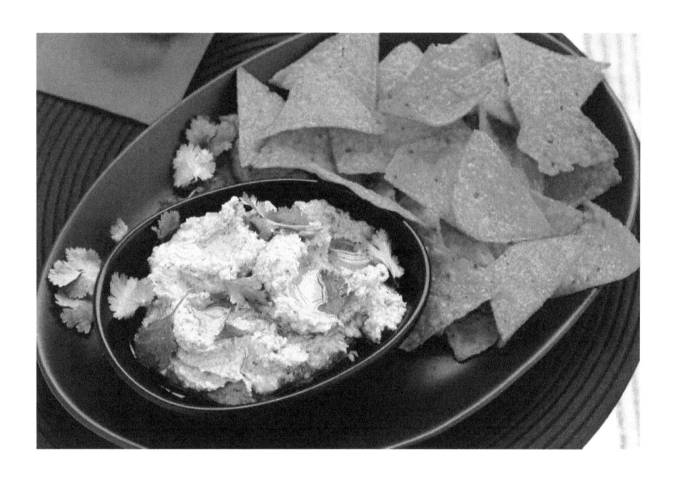

QUIRCK BREAD SAMOSAS

Recipe that everyone loves!

MAKES 4 SERVING/ TOTAL TIME 35 MINUTE

INGREDIENTS

40ml (2 tablespoons) vegetable oil, plus extra to fry

1 small onion, finely chopped

2 garlic cloves, chopped

1 small red chili, seeded, finely chopped

350g potatoes, peeled, diced, boiled

50g frozen peas, thawed

2 teaspoons mild curry powder

2 tablespoons chopped fresh coriander

8 large slices white bread, crusts removed

Mango chutney, to serve

Raita*, to serve

Salad, to serve

METHOD

STEP 1

Heat the vegetable oil in a large frying pan over medium heat. Add the onion, garlic and chili and cook for 2 minutes. Add the potato, peas and curry powder and cook for a further 1-2 minutes, mashing together to combine. Remove from the heat, season with salt and pepper and stir in the coriander.

STEP 2

Use a rolling pin to flatten each slice of bread. Divide the filling evenly and place in the center of each piece of bread. Brush the edges with a little water then fold over corner to corner, pressing the edges to form a seal.

STEP 3

Heat the oil in a deep-frying pan over high heat. Add the samosas and fry until golden on both sides. Serve with mango chutney, raita and a salad.

NUTRITION VALUE

1454 KJ Energy, 11g fat, 1g saturated fat, 6g fiber, 11g protein, 47carbs.

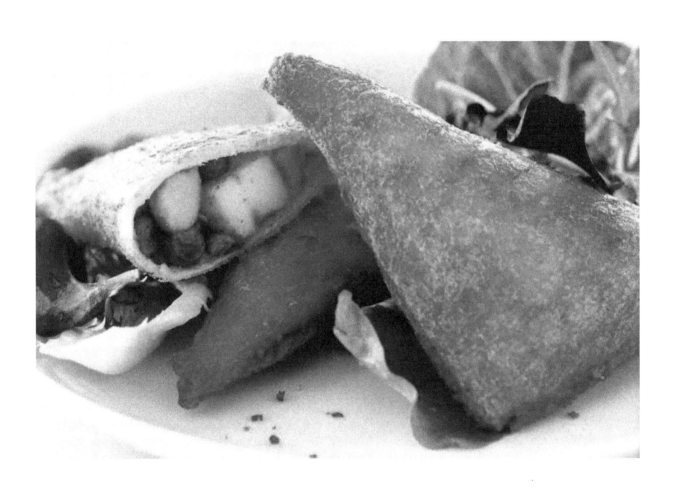

LOW-FAT PITA CRISPS

These pita crisps are a great low-fat alternative to chips or other fried snacks and crackers.

MAKES 32 SERVING/ TOTAL TIME 10 MINUTE

INGREDIENTS

4 white pita bread pockets

olive oil cooking spray

1 teaspoon paprika

METHOD

STEP 1

Preheat oven to 200°C. Spray 1 side of each pita bread with oil. Sprinkle each with 1/4 teaspoon paprika. Season with salt and pepper. Cut each bread into 8 triangles. Place, in a single layer, on 2 large baking trays.

STEP 2

Bake for 8 to 10 minutes, swapping trays after 4 minutes, or until bread is crisp. Transfer to a wire rack to cool. Serve.

NUTRITION VALUE

97 KJ Energy,
1protein, 4g carbs.

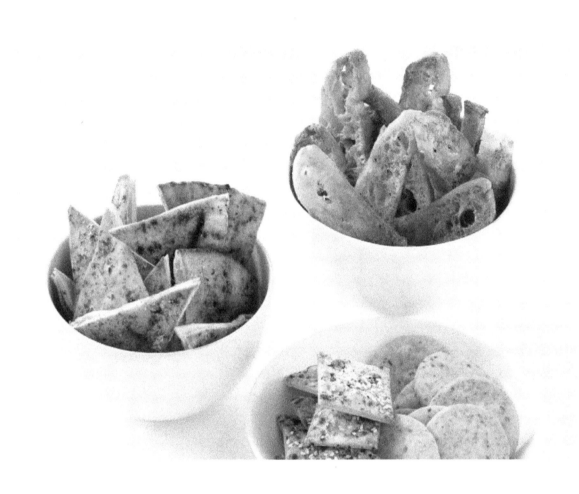

ENERGY BALLS

Energy balls, a delicious, simple, and naturally sweet snack! They're healthy, perfect to eat on the go, and ready in just 20 minutes with 4 ingredients.

MAKES 18 SERVING/ TOTAL TIME 20 MINUTE

INGREDIENTS

1 cup roasted hazelnuts (140 g)

1 1/2 cup Medjool dates (300 g)

2 tbsp unsweetened cocoa powder

1 tbsp coconut oil

METHOD

STEP 1

Place the hazelnuts in a food processor or a powerful blender and blend until they have a crumbly texture. Add the dates, cocoa powder, and coconut oil, and blend again.

STEP 2

Make the balls with your hands. I made 18 of them. Serve them with a glass of plant milk, such as oat milk, soy milk, and cashew milk, among others.

You can store them in a sealed container in the fridge for about 2 weeks or freeze them for up to 3 months.

NUTRITION VALUE

104 KJ Energy, 5.6g fat, 1.1g saturated fat, 2.3g fiber, 1.7g protein, 14.1g carbs.

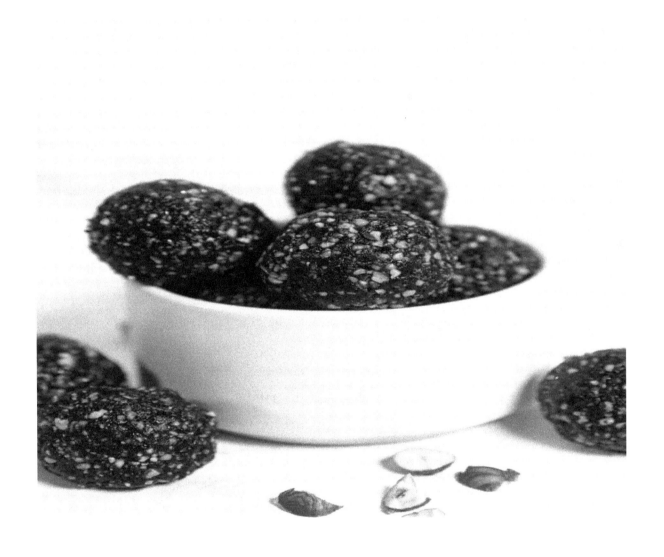

BARBECUED CAPSICUM AND BEAN SALAD

Add this lively capsicum salad to your barbecue feast for easy summer entertaining.

MAKES 4 SERVING/ TOTAL TIME 25 MINUTE

INGREDIENTS

80g (1/2 cup) pepitas (pumpkin seed kernels)

1 x 175g punnet Vine Sweet Minicaps baby capsicums, halved lengthways, deseeded

Olive oil spray

250g green beans, topped

100g baby spinach leaves

2 tablespoons balsamic vinegar

2 tablespoons extra-virgin olive oil

Pinch of sugar

Salt & freshly ground black pepper

METHOD

STEP 1

Cook the pepitas in a large frying pan over medium heat, stirring often, for 2-3 minutes, Transfer to a plate lined with paper towel. Lightly spray both sides of the baby capsicums with olive oil spray. Preheat a barbecue grill or char grill pan on medium-high. Add the baby capsicums and cook for 2-3 minutes each side or until tender and slightly charred. Transfer to a large bowl.

STEP 2

Meanwhile, cook the beans in a medium saucepan of boiling water for 3-4 minutes or until bright green and tender crisp. Refresh under cold running water. Drain well. Add the pepitas, beans and baby spinach leaves to the capsicums and gently toss until well combined.

STEP 3

Whisk together the vinegar, oil and sugar in a small jug until well combined. Taste and season with salt and pepper. Place the salad in a large serving bowl. Drizzle with the dressing and gently toss to combine. Serve immediately.

NUTRITION VALUE

938 KJ Energy, 19g fat, 3g saturated fat, 8g protein, 7g carbs.

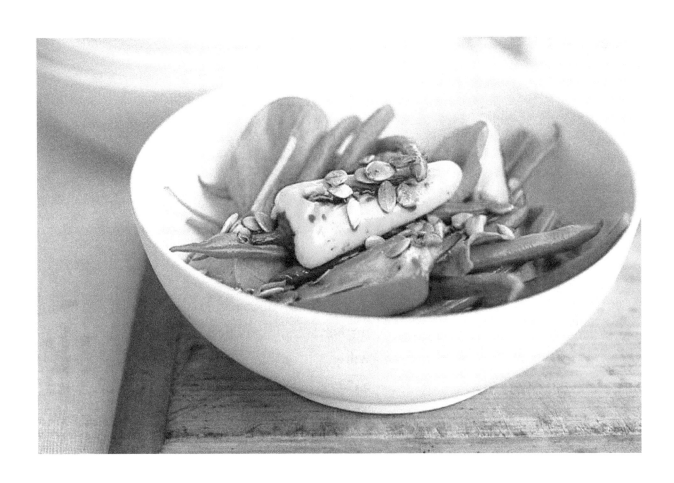

QUICK GADO

Recipe that everyone loves!

MAKES 4 SERVING/ TOTAL TIME 16 MINUTE

INGREDIENTS

1/3 cup (80ml) satay sauce

150ml light coconut milk

4 chat potatoes, cut into 1cm-thick slices

1 large carrot, peeled, sliced on the diagonal

150g baby green beans, trimmed

150g firm tofu, cut into small cubes

1/2 Chinese cabbage, shredded

200g bean sprouts

1 long red chili, thinly sliced on the diagonal, to serve

METHOD

STEP 1

Stir the satay and coconut milk together in a small saucepan over low heat, then keep warm over a very low heat.

STEP 2

Meanwhile, place the potatoes in a large steamer and steam for 3 minutes. Add the carrot and beans and steam for a further minute.

STEP 3

Add the tofu, cabbage and bean sprouts and steam for a further 1-2 minutes, or until the cabbage has just wilted.

STEP 4

To serve, divide the steamed vegetables and tofu between 4 serving plates, drizzle with the satay coconut sauce and garnish with chopped chili.

NUTRITION VALUE

1089 KJ Energy, 13g fat, 7g saturated fat, 11g protein, 21g carbs.

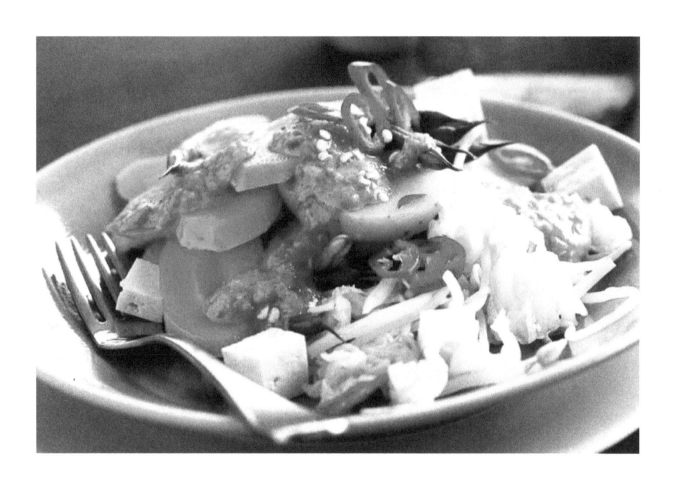

Desserts

VEGAN WAFFLES

Vegan waffles, delicious, fluffy and crispy on the outside, but soft on the inside. Add fresh fruit, maple syrup or your favorite toppings.

MAKES 3 SERVING/ TOTAL TIME 25 MINUTE

INGREDIENTS

2 cups whole wheat flour (240 g)

1/4 cup brown, cane or coconut sugar (45 g or 4 tbsp)

1 tbsp baking powder

1/2 tsp salt

1 and 1/2 cups unsweetened plant milk of your choice (375 ml), I used soy milk

1/3 cup oil of your choice (85 ml), I used melted coconut oil

2 flax eggs

2 tsp vanilla extract (optional)

METHOD

STEP 1

Add the dry ingredients to a large mixing bowl (flour, sugar, baking powder and salt) and mix until well combined.

Add all the remaining ingredients (milk, oil, flax eggs and vanilla extract) and whisk until well combined.

Preheat the waffle maker according to manufacturer's directions and spray it with oil (unless your waffle iron is non-stick).

STEP 2

Pour the recommended amount of batter onto the waffle maker and cook according to manufacturer's instructions, until golden brown on both sides. My waffles are usually ready in 3-5 minutes.

Serve with your favorite toppings. I topped my waffles with some fresh blueberries, chopped pistachios and maple syrup, but they're also delicious with some vegan butter on top.

Keep leftovers in an airtight container for about 3 days in the fridge or 1 month in the freezer.

NUTRITION VALUE

339 KJ Energy, 17.7g fat, 13.9g saturated fat, 6.8g fiber, 9g protein, 39g carbs.

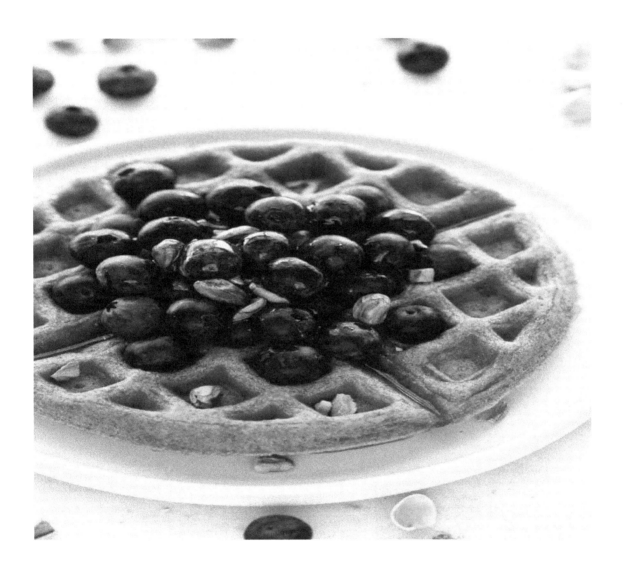

VEGAN HOT CHOCOLATE

Vegan hot chocolate, a delicious plant-based drink that everyone loves. It's sweet and creamy, it needs just 4 ingredients and only takes 10 minutes!

MAKES 2 SERVING/ TOTAL TIME 10 MINUTE

INGREDIENTS

2 cups unsweetened plant milk (500 ml), I used almond milk

2/3 cup vegan chocolate chips (120 g)

1 tbsp sugar, I used cane sugar

1 tsp vanilla extract, optional

METHOD

STEP 1

Add all the ingredients to a saucepan and cook over medium heat until the chocolate is completely melted, stirring occasionally. Serve immediately

NUTRITION VALUE

180 KJ Energy, 8.8g fat, 4.5g saturated fat, 2.3g fiber, 2.8g protein, 20.5g carbs.

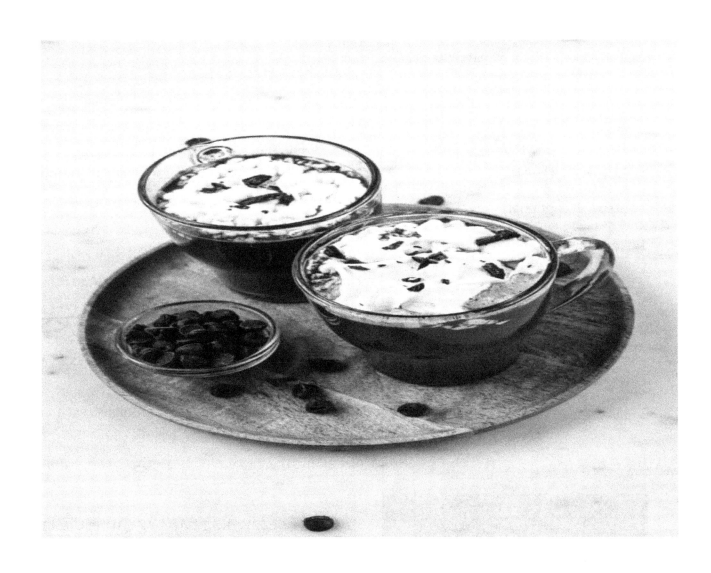

VEGAN CHOCOLATE CHIP COOKIES

Vegan chocolate chip cookies, perfect for everyday baking and made with 9 ingredients. They are so crisp on the outside, but soft and chewy on the inside.

MAKES 24 SERVING/ TOTAL TIME 30 MINUTE

INGREDIENTS

2 and 1/2 cup whole wheat flour (375 g)

1 cup brown, cane or coconut sugar (180 g)

1/2 tsp baking soda

1/4 tsp salt (optional)

1/2 cup unsweetened plant milk of your choice (125 ml), I used soy milk

1/4 cup coconut oil (65 ml), melted

2 flax eggs

1 tsp vanilla extract (optional)

3/4 cup vegan chocolate chips (130 g)

METHOD

STEP 1

Preheat the oven to 350ºF or 180ºC.

Combine the dry ingredients in a large mixing bowl (flour, sugar, baking soda and salt).

Add the liquid ingredients to the large mixing bowl (milk, oil, flax eggs and vanilla extract) and stir until well combined.

STEP 2

Add the chocolate chips and stir until they're evenly incorporated. Refrigerate the dough for about 30 minutes. Now it's time to make your cookies Press down slightly to flatten. Bake for about 15 minutes or until the cookies are golden at the edges, but still a little underdone in the center.

Remove from the oven and let the cookies rest on the hot baking sheet for at least 5 minutes before transferring them to a cooling rack or a serving plate.

NUTRITION VALUE

132 KJ Energy, 4.3g fat, 3.2g saturated fat, 2.1g fiber, 2.6g protein, 22.1g carbs.

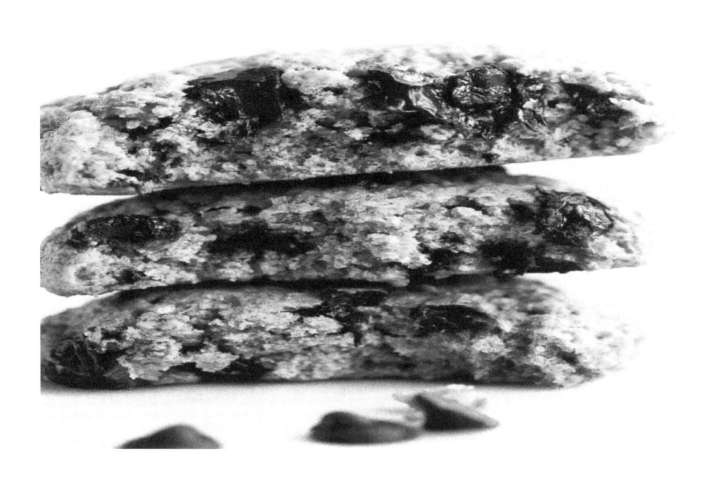

SIMPLE VEGAN BANANA BREAD

This is the best vegan banana bread ever! Sweet, moist in the inside, crispy on the outside, and full of flavor. Perfect for breakfast or dessert.

MAKES 12 SERVING/ TOTAL TIME 70 MINUTE

INGREDIENTS

1 and 1/2 cups mashed very ripe bananas (about 3 large bananas)

2 cups whole wheat flour (240 g)

3/4 cup brown, cane or coconut sugar (135 g)

1 tsp ground cinnamon

1 tsp baking soda

1/4 tsp salt

1 flax egg

1/2 cup unsweetened plant milk of your choice (125 ml), I used soy milk

1/3 cup coconut oil (85 ml), melted

1 tsp vanilla extract, optional

METHOD

STEP 1

Preheat the oven to 350°F or 180ºC with an oven rack in the bottom third of the oven. Mash the bananas with a fork and set aside. Add the dry ingredients to a large mixing bowl and mix until well combined.

Add all the remaining ingredients (mashed bananas, flax egg, oil and vanilla extract). Stir until well mixed. Line a 9×5-inch (23×13 cm) loaf pan with parchment paper or grease it with some coconut oil.

STEP 2

Add the batter to the pan and bake for 60 to 70 minutes Stick a toothpick into the center of the loaf and if it comes out clean, the loaf is done. Cover the top with foil if the banana bread gets browned, but the middle isn't done yet.

Let it cool for 15 minutes on the loaf pan before transferring it to a cooling rack and then let it cool completely.

NUTRITION VALUE

204 KJ Energy, 8g fat, 7g saturated fat, 3.7g fiber, 3.7g protein, 31.7g carbs.

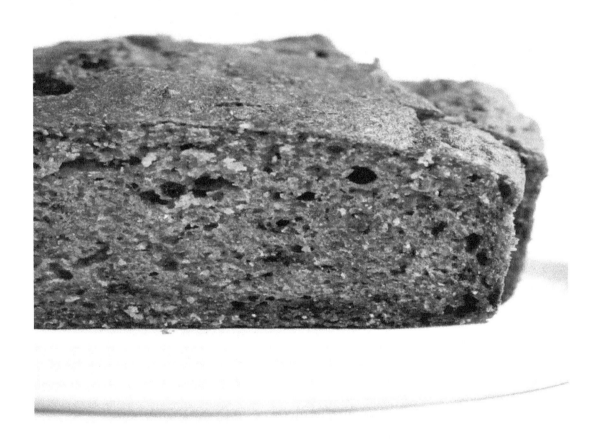

VEGAN CHOCOLATE COOKIES

Vegan chocolate cookies, the best vegan cookies in the whole world. They're thick, soft and fudgy and made with just 9 simple ingredients.

MAKES 18 SERVING/ TOTAL TIME 15 MINUTE

INGREDIENTS

1/2 cup coconut oil (105 g), solid, not melted, see notes

3/4 cup brown, cane or coconut sugar (135 g)

1 tsp vanilla extract (optional)

3/4 cup unsweetened plant milk of your choice (190 ml), I used soy milk

1/2 cup unsweetened cocoa powder (40 g)

1 tsp baking soda

1/4 tsp salt

1 and 3/4 cups whole wheat flour (210 g)

1/2 cup vegan chocolate chips (90 g) + 2 tbsp for topping your cookies, (optional),

METHOD

STEP 1

Preheat the oven to 350ºF or 180ºC.

Add the coconut oil and the sugar to a bowl and mash them with a fork until well combined. You'll get a creamy mixture, with no coconut oil chunks.

Add the vanilla extract, milk and cocoa powder. Mix until well combined.

Add the baking soda and salt and mix again.

If the temperature is warm where you are, chill the mixture in the fridge for 15-30 minutes to firm up,

STEP 2

Add the flour and stir again. Then add the chocolate chips and stir until just combined (don't over stir).

Make balls with your hands, place them onto a lined baking sheet, press them down a little bit and evenly distribute them, about 2 inches or 5 cm apart because the cookies will expand in the oven

Let them cool for 5 minutes on the baking sheet before transferring them to a cooling rack and then let them cool completely.

NUTRITION VALUE	157 KJ Energy, 8.2g fat, 6.7g saturated fat, 2.7g fiber, 2.9g protein, 8.2g carbs.

VEGAN BREAD PUDDING

Vegan bread pudding, a delicious dessert, so easy to make and only requires 7 simple ingredients. It's perfect served with sugar glaze or ice cream.

MAKES 8 SERVING/ TOTAL TIME 1 HOUR 20 MINUTE

INGREDIENTS

1 pound stale vegan bread of your choice, cut into cubes (450 g), I used spelt bread

3 cups unsweetened plant milk of your choice (750 ml), I used soy milk

3/4 cup brown, cane or coconut sugar (150 g)

1/4 cup flax seeds (4 tbsp)

1 tbsp coconut oil (optional)

1 tsp vanilla extract (optional)

1/2 tsp ground cinnamon

METHOD

STEP 1

Place the bread cubes in a large mixing bowl and set aside.

Add the rest of the ingredients to a blender and blend until smooth.

Pour the mixture all over the bread, stir and set aside for about 1 hour at room temperature.

Preheat the oven to 350ºF or 180ºC.

STEP 2

Place the pudding mixture in a 9×9-inch (22×22 cm) baking dish and bake for 60 to 70 minutes or until the bread pudding is golden brown on the outside and cooked on the inside. Baking time may vary depending on your oven, my pudding was ready in 70 minutes. If the pudding is golden brown, but uncooked, cover with some aluminum foil and cook until is ready.

Remove from the oven and allow to cool slightly before serving. You can also enjoy it cold (I actually think it's better the next day). I added some brown sugar glaze on top, but it's optional.

NUTRITION VALUE

263 KJ Energy, 6.8g fat, 1.8g saturated fat, 3.2g fiber, 8.6 protein, 45.3g carbs.

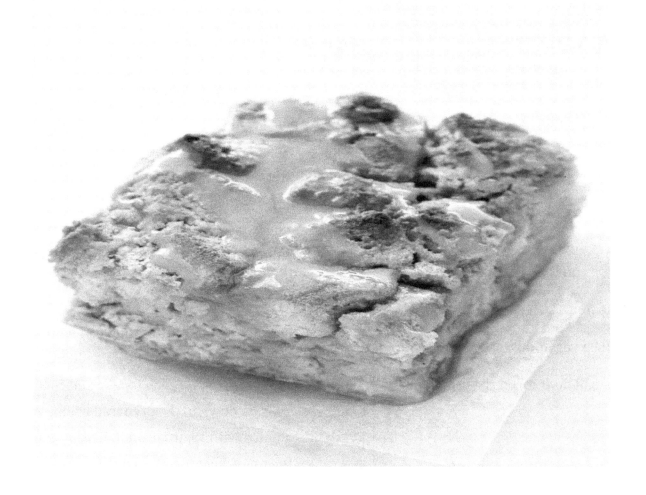

VEGAN APPLE PIE TAQUITOS

Vegan apple pie taquitos, a delicious, crispy and sweet dessert. They're stuffed with an amazing apple pie filling and baked instead of fried.

MAKES 5 SERVING/ TOTAL TIME 45 MINUTE

INGREDIENTS

Coconut oil (optional)

2 Granny Smith apples, peeled, cored and diced

3 tbsp + 1 tsp brown sugar, divided

1/2 + 1/8 tsp ground cinnamon, divided

1/2 tsp vanilla extract (optional)

2 tbsp flour, I used brown rice flour

1/4 tbsp vegan caramel sauce (65 ml)

5–6 small flour tortillas, I used 5

METHOD

STEP 1

Preheat the oven to 375ºF or 190ºC.

Heat 1 tbsp of coconut oil in a skillet and add the apples, 3 tbsp of brown sugar and 1/2 tsp of ground cinnamon. Stir and cook over medium-high heat for about 5 minutes, stirring occasionally.

Add the vanilla extract and flour, stir and cook for 1 minute. Add the vegan caramel sauce, stir and remove from the heat.

STEP 2

Grease an 8×8-inch (20×20 cm) baking pan with some coconut oil and set aside. Divide the apple filling among 5 tortillas and tightly roll up each tortilla . Place the taquitos seam-side down in the prepared baking pan. Brush the taquitos with some coconut oil (optional) and add some cinnamon sugar on top. To make the cinnamon sugar, add 1 tsp of brown sugar and 1/8 tsp of ground cinnamon to a blender and blend until you get a powdered texture. Bake for 25 minutes or until golden brown.

Serve immediately and add more vegan caramel sauce on top (optional).

NUTRITION VALUE

341 KJ Energy, 14.7g fat, 10g saturated fat, 4.6g fiber, 2.8g protein, 51.9g carbs.

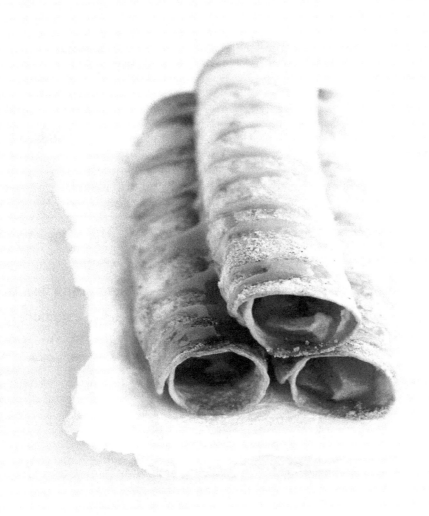

VEGAN CARAMEL SAUCE

Vegan caramel sauce, made with 3 ingredients in less than 5 minutes. This magic sauce is perfect for topping on ice cream, apple slices or any dessert.

MAKES 10 SERVING/ TOTAL TIME 5 MINUTE

INGREDIENTS

1/4 cup almond butter (4 tbsp)

1/4 cup maple syrup (4 tbsp)

2 tbsp coconut oil

1/4 tsp vanilla extract (optional)

Pinch of salt (optional)

METHOD

STEP 1

Heat the maple syrup and coconut oil in a saucepan (or in a bowl in the microwave) for 30-60 seconds or until the coconut oil is melted.

STEP 2

Add the mixture to a bowl and add the rest of the ingredients (almond butter, vanilla extract and salt). Stir until well combined. Depending on how thick is your almond butter, you'll need to add more or less, so add 2 tbsp first, stir and add more gently until you get the perfect consistency.

Enjoy this caramel sauce hot, cold, with apple slices or just use it to make any recipe that calls for caramel sauce.

Keep leftovers in a sealed container in the fridge for 1-2 weeks.

NUTRITION VALUE

48 Energy, 3.1g fat, 2.7g saturated fat, 0.1g protein, 5.4g carbs.

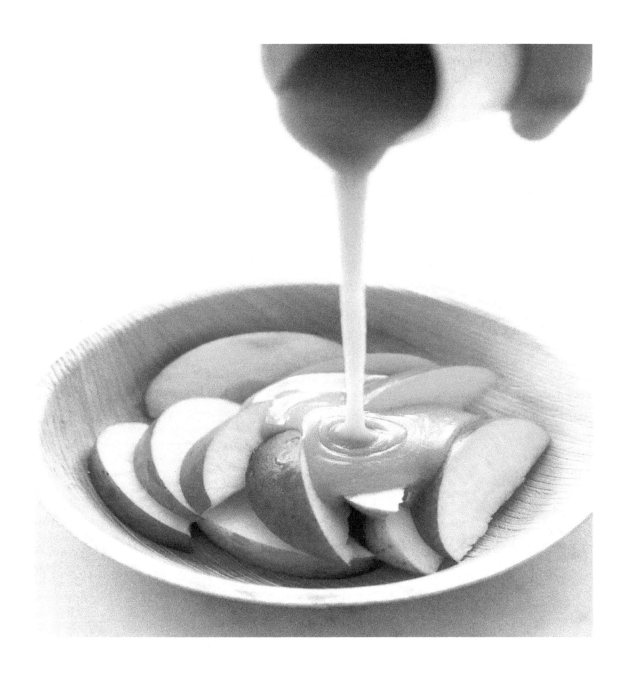

VEGAN PUMPKIN CAKE (GLUTEN FREE)

Vegan pumpkin cake, made with natural ingredients and topped with vegan cashew frosting. It's also gluten-free and the perfect dessert for fall!

MAKES 8 SERVING/ TOTAL TIME 60 MINUTE

INGREDIENTS

For the vegan pumpkin cake:

- 1/2 cup brown rice flour (70 g)
- 3/4 cup oat flour (85 g), gluten-free if needed
- 1/2 cup brown, coconut or cane sugar (1oo g)
- 1 and 1/2 tsp baking soda
- 1 tsp ground cinnamon
- 1 tsp pumpkin pie spice
- 2 flax eggs
- 1 tbsp apple cider vinegar
- 3/4 cup coconut milk (190 ml)
- 3/4 cup pumpkin puree (190 ml)

Toppings (optional):

- Vegan cashew frosting
- Chopped walnuts
- Extra ground cinnamon

METHOD

STEP 1

Preheat the oven to 400ºF or 200ºC.

Mix the dry ingredients in a large mixing bowl

Add the liquid ingredients to the mixing bowl (flax eggs, vinegar, coconut milk and pumpkin puree) and mix until well combined.

Grease the cake pan with some oil. If you use a non-stick pan, omit this step. We usually place a sheet of parchment paper on the bottom of the cake pan to avoid using oil. We used a 9 inch or 22 cm round cake pan.

STEP 2

Pour the batter into the pan and bake for about 40-45 minutes or until deep golden brown and a toothpick inserted into the center comes out clean.

Remove the cake from the oven and let it rest in the pan until completely cool.

Serve with your favorite toppings.

NUTRITION VALUE	148 Energy, 2.7g fat, 1.4g saturated fat, 2.2g fiber, 2.6g protein, 2.2g carbs.

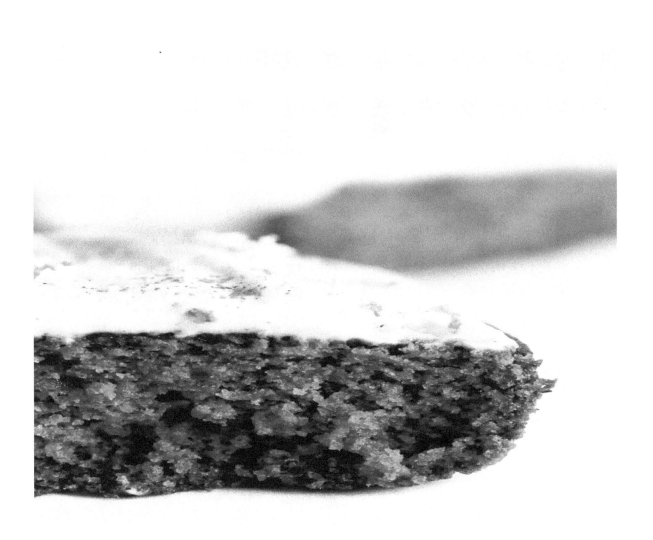

VEGAN APPLE CRISP (GLUTEN FREE)

This vegan apple crisp is also gluten-free and one of my all-time favorite fall desserts. It only requires 8 ingredients and 1 bowl!

MAKES 2 SERVING/ TOTAL TIME 55 MINUTE

INGREDIENTS

For the filling:

- 1-pound apples (450 g)
- 1/4 cup brown, coconut or cane sugar (4 tbsp or 20 g)
- 1 tbsp brown rice flour
- 1 tbsp lemon juice
- 1/2 tsp cinnamon powder
- Zest of half a lemon (optional)

For the topping:

- 1/2 cup rolled oats (50 g), gf if needed
- 1/2 cup brown rice flour (70 g)
- 1/4 cup brown, coconut or cane sugar (4 tbsp or 20 g)
- 2 tbsp coconut oil, melted, see notes for an oil-free alternative
- 1/2 tsp cinnamon powder

METHOD

STEP 1

Preheat the oven to 350ºF or 180ºC.

Peel the apples, quarter them, remove the cores, and use a paring knife to thinly slice lengthwise

Add all the filling ingredients to a large mixing bowl and mix until well combined.

Place the filling into a baking dish. We used a 9 1/4" x 6" x 2" or 23 x 15 x 5 cm baking dish, but you can use any other rectangular or square dish you want.

Add the topping ingredients to the same large mixing bowl you used to mix the filling ingredients. Then mix until well combined and add to the top of the filling in an even layer.

STEP 2

Bake for 40 minutes or until the top is golden brown. Let it cool for a while before serving. We served our apple crisp with some coconut whipped cream, but it's also delicious with ice cream or just by itself.

NUTRITION VALUE	240 Energy, 8.3g fat, 6.1g saturated fat, 3.1g fiber, 3.3g protein, 40.6g carbs.

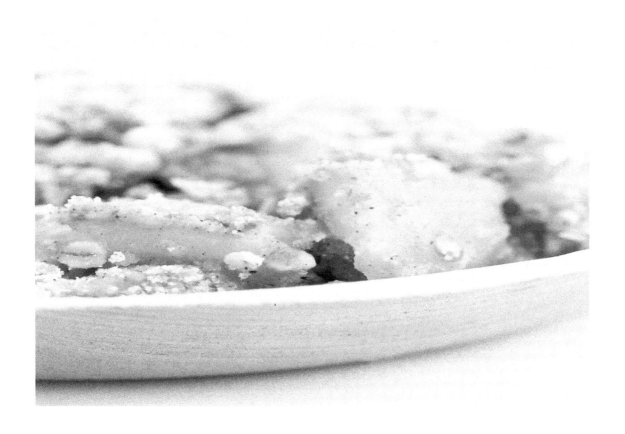

CPSIA information can be obtained
at www.ICGtesting.com
Printed in the USA
BVHW011652040521
606415BV00007B/1876